Ethan Waisberg • Joshua Ong • Andrew G. Lee
Editors

Ophthalmology of Sports

Springer

Editors
Ethan Waisberg
Department of Clinical Neurosciences
University of Cambridge
Cambridge, UK

Joshua Ong
Department of Ophthalmology
and Visual Sciences
University of Michigan Kellogg Eye Center
Ann Arbor, MI, USA

Andrew G. Lee
Department of Ophthalmology
Blanton Eye Institute, Houston Methodist
Hospital
Houston, TX, USA

ISBN 978-3-031-88644-7 ISBN 978-3-031-88645-4 (eBook)
https://doi.org/10.1007/978-3-031-88645-4

This Springer imprint is published by the registered company Springer Nature Switzerland AG
The registered company address is: Gewerbestrasse 11, 6330 Cham, Switzerland

Preface

Ever tried catching a football with blurry vision? Or dodging opponents when your peripheral vision is failing you? In sports, vision is not just about seeing clearly, it's about reacting, tracking, and consistently staying one step ahead. *Ophthalmology of Sports* dives into the fascinating world where peak athletic performance meets vision science.

From cutting-edge vision training, to high-speed ocular injuries, this textbook explores how athletes can gain a competitive edge by enhancing their vision and by protecting their eyes. Whether you are an ophthalmologist, competitive athlete, or just a fan that loves the vision science behind the game, this textbook is for you.

Each chapter includes contributions from experts who have directly worked with elite athletes across major sporting leagues, including the NBA, NHL, NCAA, Formula 1, NFL, ATP, and the Olympics. These experts share invaluable real-world insights, the latest research, and practical tips to elevate athletic performance.

As baseball legend Ted Williams once said, "You can't hit what you can't see." Vision can be the difference between winning and losing, between a missed opportunity and a championship winning play.

Whether it's the final lap of the Grand Prix, or a game-winning buzzer-beater, great vision is the secret weapon driving success in all sports.

Let's see the game like never before!

Cambridge, UK — Ethan Waisberg

Ann Arbor, MI, USA — Joshua Ong

Houston, TX, USA — Andrew G. Lee

Acknowledgments

Dr. Ethan Waisberg
I would like to express my deepest gratitude to my parents, Jennifer and Darrell, for their constant belief and unwavering support throughout this journey. A special thank you to my brother, Cooper, whose passion for sports has always been an inspiration. Growing up with my brother and playing competitive hockey and tennis together not only created unforgettable memories but sparked my interest in the connection between vision and athletic performance.

This book is dedicated to you, my greatest supporters and lifelong inspiration.

Dr. Joshua Ong
I would like to acknowledge and dedicate this book to my loving family. As a son, brother, and grandson to a family that has always emphasized a healthy and active lifestyle, I find it very gratifying to dedicate this book to you all. I would like to thank my parents, Dennis Ong and Timmy Ong, for being my role models. Thank you for all your support and love, it means the world to me. I am particularly grateful for your early and constant encouragement to live an active lifestyle and reminisce the days of going together to the local basketball gym to practice shooting three-pointers or playing tennis together. To my dad, I am still always in awe that you swim nearly every single day, even when you're traveling to multiple states or countries. To my mom, I always appreciated your proactive effort to incorporate various sports into our lives, from tetherball to indoor basketball hoops. I would like to thank my siblings, Jeremiah Ong and Hannah Ong. Thank you for being absolutely dependable and incredible lifelong friends. As I have told many, both of you have demonstrated time and time again that you are able to quickly pick up various sports and excel at a high level. I hope you both find the contents of this book interesting as it highlights the connection of vision and sports performance. I would like to thank my grandmother, Shu Mei Wong. I am always inspired by your dedication to an active lifestyle and thank you again for giving me your favorite table tennis paddle many years ago! Lastly, I'd like to express my deepest gratitude to my late grandfather, Tak Hin Lee. Thank you for everything, grandpa.

Dr. Andrew G. Lee

Dr. Lee wishes to recognize and thank his mentors in neuro-ophthalmology: his fellowship director (1993) at the Wilmer Eye Institute, Johns Hopkins Hospital, Neil Miller, MD; his colleagues and best friends, Tony Arnold, MD, at UCLA, and Paul Brazis, MD, at Mayo Clinic, for their invaluable guidance, mentorship, and friendship over the past 30 years. He thanks his parents, Alberto C. Lee, MD, and Rosalind G. Lee, MD, for their unwavering support and love and for instilling in him a love of science, intellectual curiosity, and a passion for teaching and learning. Dr. Lee is also grateful to his siblings, Amy Lee, MD, and Richard Lee, for being critical sources of advice and counsel and years of nerd fun. He is especially appreciative of his (now grown) daughters, Rachael Lee and Virginia Lee, for reminding their father every day what life is about. Most of all, Dr. Lee thanks his loving and lovely wife, Hilary Beaver, MD, who remains his vibrant muse, tireless inspiration, and tolerant soul mate over 35 years of marriage.

Book Cover Artwork Acknowledgment

Conceptualization and production of the artwork cover for this book, Ophthalmology of Sports, was done by Joshua Ong, MD, and Hamza Memon.

Contents

About the Editors

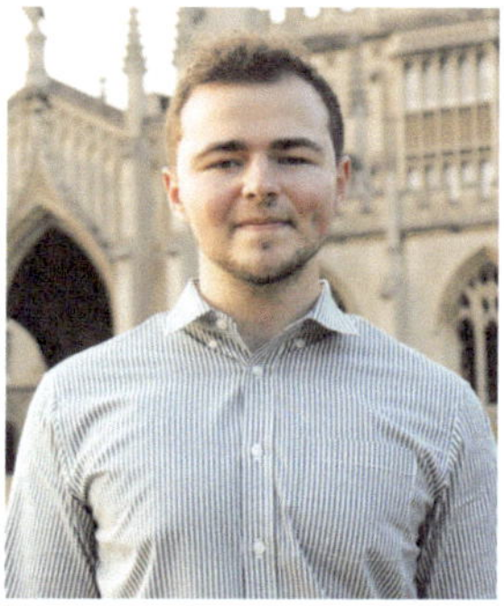

Ethan Waisberg is an Academic Foundation Doctor at the University of Cambridge. His research interests in ophthalmology are varied and range from eye health in extreme environments such as spaceflight with NASA astronauts, to the role of ocular performance in athletic competitions.

Dr. Waisberg helped develop a virtual-reality (VR) headset to perform various visual assessments on NASA astronauts during long-duration spaceflight that will be used on future NASA missions. His research has led to massive developments in the understanding of Spaceflight Associated Neuro-Ocular Syndrome (SANS), a condition that affects nearly 75% of astronauts, and is crucial to fully understand this condition prior to the mission to Mars. Dr. Waisberg's research has been presented at major global forums, including The White House, United Nations, and World Health Organization and has been featured in international media such as the BBC, NY Post and The Times. Beyond medicine, Dr. Waisberg is an avid ice hockey and tennis player, having proudly represented the University of Cambridge in both sports. He was named Player of the Match in the historic Cambridge vs. Oxford Varsity Ice Hockey Match and his firsthand experience as an athlete has deepened his understanding of the physiological and visual demands in high-performance sports.

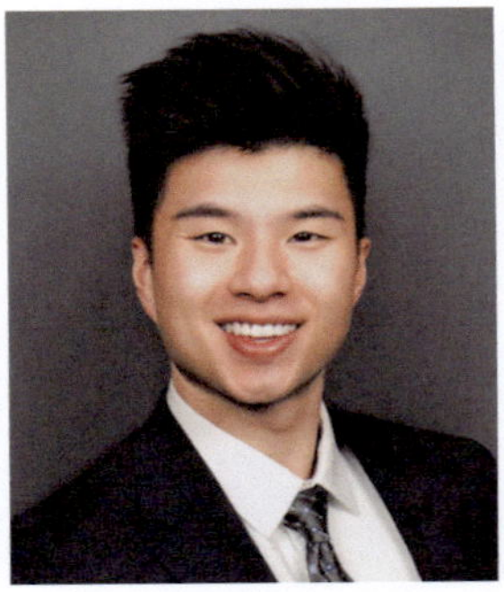

Joshua Ong is an Ophthalmology Resident Physician at the Department of Ophthalmology and Visual Sciences, University of Michigan Kellogg Eye Center. He completed his MD degree at the University of Pittsburgh School of Medicine, graduating top of his class in medical research where he was awarded the O'Malley Award for Outstanding Medical Student Research for his NASA-funded research in space medicine ophthalmology. He was the 2025 recipient of The Paul R. Lichter Resident Mentor Award. He served as Associate Editor for the textbook "Spaceflight Associated Neuro-ocular Syndrome" and his areas of interest include space medicine ophthalmology including ocular surface risks in space and spaceflight associated neuro-ocular syndrome (SANS), as well as technology development to optimize detection of irreversible but preventable causes of blindness.

Dr. Ong's work includes including conducting research on a NASA-funded tissue engineering project that launched into space and artificial intelligence frameworks for SANS. He placed 2nd place at NASA's space medicine conference for his work on augmented reality to counteract damaged astronaut vision on the anticipated mission to Mars. His work in artificial intelligence to further understand SANS has been presented at the United Nations (UN) and World Health Organization (WHO) at the UN/WHO International Conference on Space and Global Health with the goal to contribute toward recommendations for the UN General Assembly Resolution on Space and Global Health. He has also conducted and published vision science research in collaboration with the National Football League (NFL) with the goal of optimizing accuracy and precision for NFL official on-field decision making. Dr. Ong delivered a TEDx Talk in 2025 discussing his journey in space medicine and the applications of these novel technologies to address barriers to vision care for marginalized communities.

Dr. Ong serves in various editorial roles in scientific journals and as a reviewer for various high-impact scientific journals in ophthalmology and space medicine. He has authored over 200 publications in peer-reviewed journals and book chapters. Dr. Joshua Ong was listed in Forbes 30 Under 30 for his work.

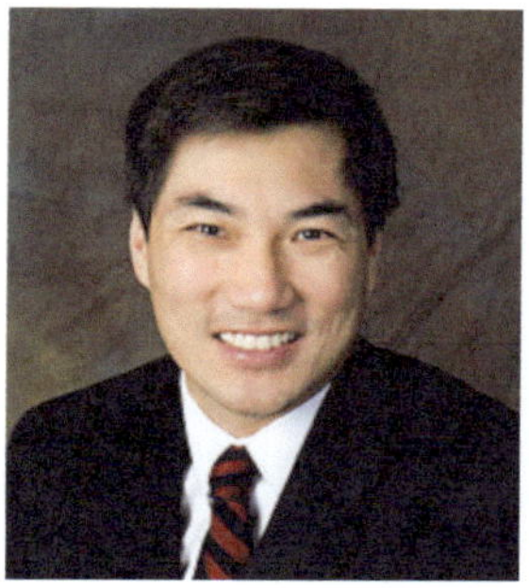

Andrew G. Lee is the Herb and Jean Lyman Centennial Chair in Ophthalmology and is the Founding Chairman of the Blanton Eye Institute, Department of Ophthalmology at Houston Methodist Hospital in Houston, Texas. He is Professor of Ophthalmology, Neurology, and Neurosurgery at Weill Cornell Medicine; an Adjunct Professor of Ophthalmology at Baylor College of Medicine, Texas A and M College of Medicine, University of Iowa, and the University of Buffalo; and Clinical Professor at the University of Texas Medical Branch (UTMB) in Galveston, Texas, and the UT MD Anderson Cancer Center.

He is a graduate of the University of Virginia (UVA) undergraduate and UVA School of Medicine. He was an ophthalmology resident and chief resident at Baylor College of Medicine and a clinical neuro-ophthalmology fellow and Fight for Sight postdoctoral research fellow at the Wilmer Eye Institute, the Johns Hopkins Hospital.

Dr. Lee has served in numerous leadership roles at the American Academy of Ophthalmology (AAO) and has received the AAO Achievement Award, Senior Achievement Award, Secretariat Award (three times), and Lifetime Achievement Award. He is a past President, a past Chairman of the Board, and Senior VP for Advocacy of the North American Neuro-ophthalmology Society.

Dr. Lee has received the teaching award 15 times at 7 different academic institutions including the Osler Excellence in Teaching Award, the Baylor College of Medicine Dan B. Jones Teaching Award, University of Iowa Charles Phelps Award, the Texas A and M Mid Career Education award, the HMH Presidential Excellence in Education, and the Houston Methodist Hospital Sherilynn Gordon Memorial Leadership Award.

Dr. Lee has been the invited speaker at over 400 national and international medical meetings; has written over 600 peer-reviewed publications and 14 full text-books; and has given 15 named lectures. His h-index is 68 and his i-10 is 367 with over 18,000 citations. He has been named one of top 30 ophthalmologists in the United States by *Newsweek* magazine and is the only neuro-ophthalmologist on the list.

He lives in Houston, Texas, with his wife, Hilary; his two daughters (Rachael and Virginia); and his two cats (Lola and Miss Kitty).

Chapter 1
Ophthalmology of Basketball

Yannie Guo, Joshua Ong, Ethan Waisberg, Andrew G. Lee, Rod Foroozan, Terry Kim, C. Ellis Wisely, and Michael T. Yen

1.1 Introduction

Basketball is one of the most popular sports globally. Full of dynamic player movements and flying projectiles, it is also the leading cause of sports-related ophthalmic injuries [1, 2]. While many of these injuries are self-limited and may not result in significant visual impairment [3], it is important to identify the wide range of ophthalmic injuries that can arise from playing basketball and how such injuries can be

Author, Andrew G. Lee, MD, discloses that he has served or is serving as a consultant for the following companies: AstraZeneca, Alexion, Bristol Mayers Squibb, National Football League, Catalyst, Viridian, Ethyreal, NASA, US Department of Justice, Dompe, and Stoke.

Y. Guo (✉)
School of Medicine, Baylor College of Medicine, Houston, TX, USA
e-mail: Yannie.Guo@bcm.edu

J. Ong
Department of Ophthalmology and Visual Sciences, University of Michigan Kellogg Eye Center, Ann Arbor, MI, USA

E. Waisberg
Department of Clinical Neurosciences, University of Cambridge, Cambridge, UK

A. G. Lee
Department of Ophthalmology, Blanton Eye Institute, Houston Methodist Hospital, Houston, TX, USA

R. Foroozan · M. T. Yen
Department of Ophthalmology, Cullen Eye Institute, Baylor College of Medicine, Houston, TX, USA

T. Kim · C. E. Wisely
Department of Ophthalmology, Duke Eye Center, Duke University School of Medicine, Durham, NC, USA

E. Waisberg et al. (eds.), *Ophthalmology of Sports*,
https://doi.org/10.1007/978-3-031-88645-4_1

managed in order to minimize long-term consequences. In this chapter, we review the epidemiology of basketball-related ophthalmic injuries, highlight some common injuries that arise, and describe countermeasure strategies that players can take to minimize their risk of experiencing such injuries while playing basketball. Finally, while there are several potential mechanisms of visual impairment from basketball-related injuries, we also discuss potential strategies of visual training that may improve performance as well as visuomotor benefits that a player may gain from playing basketball.

1.2 Ocular Trauma

1.2.1 Epidemiology

Due to the high frequency of physical contact between players and the immense popularity of the sport, basketball is the leading cause of sports-related injuries in general and specifically sports-related eye injuries [4]. Emergency departments in the United States have evaluated 30,000 patients with sports-related ocular trauma each year, with basketball as the cause of over 20% of these cases for all ages [3, 5]. Most individuals were male and under the age of 18 years [6]. Among US college athletes, it was found that men's and women's basketball had the top two rates of ocular injury per playtime out of any collegiate sport [7].

Ocular trauma due to basketball is extremely common. Thus, it is important that courtside medical personnel, emergency department healthcare workers, and other members of the medical field are aware of the various types of eye injuries that arise from basketball as well as how to assess and manage them.

Through an investigation using the National Electronic Injury Surveillance System (NEISS) database from 2012 through 2021, over 90% of eye injuries from playing basketball were found to be caused by direct player-player contact [6]. This is further supported by an investigation into national databases of high school and NCAA college athletes, which identified eye injury rates to be higher in competition than in practice [8]. From these epidemiological studies, corneal abrasions were identified as the most common basketball-related eye injury in both children and adults [6]. Other common eye injuries include eyelid lacerations, orbital fractures, and traumatic iritis [9]. We discuss details of these as well as other common basketball-related eye injuries in the next section.

1.2.2 Common Eye Injuries

While there are numerous mechanisms causing eye or periorbital injuries as a result of playing basketball, most arise from player contact with another player (e.g., fingers, elbows) rather than player contact with the basketball itself [6, 10]. In this section, we discuss a few of the most common basketball-related eye injuries along with treatment regimens, indications for returning to play, and considerations for short- and long-term consequences.

1.2.2.1 Corneal Abrasion and Extraocular Foreign Body

The most common ocular injury resulting from basketball in both children and adults is a corneal abrasion [6]. The cornea is the outermost structure of the eye that lies just anterior to the anterior chamber and functions to refract light rays that travel toward the retina [11]. A corneal abrasion occurs when the outermost layer of the cornea, the epithelium, is scratched or scraped.

Clinical Findings and Diagnosis

Corneal abrasion is often associated with symptoms of sharp eye pain and irritation, tearing, difficulty opening the eye, photophobia, conjunctival injection, and decreased visual acuity [12]. At the courtside, a suspected corneal abrasion can be initially assessed by inspecting the eye and eyelids with a penlight for corneal defects, the presence of a foreign body, evidence of penetrating trauma, and to exclude intraocular injury. If the presence of a foreign body is suspected, the examination will involve eversion of the upper eyelid to expose any retained material (Fig. 1.1) [13]. Diagnosis of a corneal abrasion can be further confirmed via topical fluorescein staining, which may indicate the presence and extent of an abrasion when observed under cobalt blue light by highlighting areas of denuded corneal epithelium (Fig. 1.2) [14].

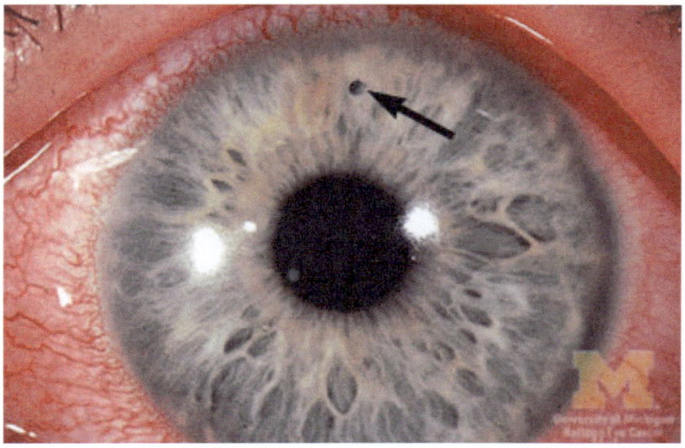

Fig. 1.1 An extraocular (corneal) foreign body causing foreign body sensation and eye inflammation. (Source: Image from the University of Michigan Kellogg Eye Center and reprinted with permission from Dr. Jonathan D. Trobe, MD (https://kellogg.umich.edu/theeyeshaveit/trauma/corneal_foreign_body.html) under Creative Commons Attribution 3.0 License)

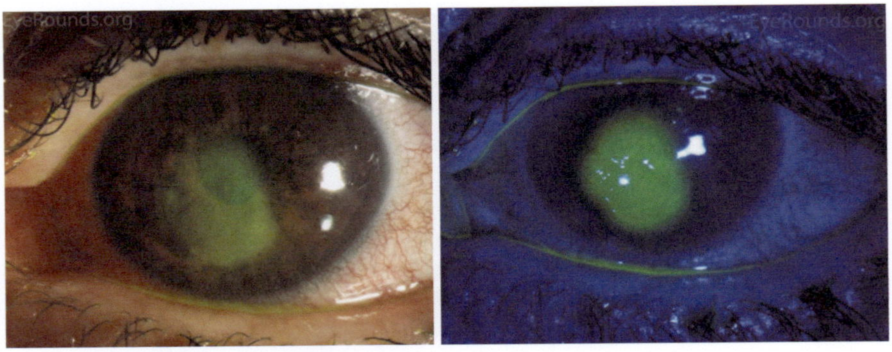

Fig. 1.2 A corneal abrasion after the application of fluorescein dye under white light (left) and under cobalt blue light (right). (Source: Image from EyeRounds.org, The University of Iowa and reprinted with permission from Dr. Jesse Vislisel, MD (https://webeye.ophth.uiowa.edu/eyeforum/atlas/pages/corneal-abrasion/index.htm#gsc.tab=0) under Creative Commons License (https://creativecommons.org/licenses/by-nc-nd/3.0/deed.en))

Treatment

The goals of treatment for a corneal abrasion include removal of any foreign body, relief of symptoms, and prevention of complications such as infection. Common treatment options include ocular lubrication, topical cycloplegic agents, and topical antibiotics. Oral and topical analgesics (e.g., non-steroidal anti-inflammatory drugs (NSAIDs)), are typically used for pain control, but more severe cases may require opioid medications. Topical anesthetics, however, should be used judiciously as excessive use can lead to delayed healing and worsening keratopathy [14, 15]. An ocular surface foreign body can be removed by everting the eyelids and flushing the eye with sterile saline or with a cotton swab. Instances in which the foreign body is embedded in the cornea or otherwise difficult to remove may require the use of a tool such as a bent small (27 gauge) needle tip [16].

Return to Play

Immediate return to play after a minor eye injury is relatively common if the patient does not experience any symptoms or discomfort and after any superficial, non-penetrating foreign body is removed. If symptoms persist however, there is the short-term option of using a bandage contact lens to relieve symptoms and expedite return to play [13]. Prolonged use of topical anesthetics may be toxic to the corneal epithelium and thus should be avoided [17]. Relative contraindications to immediate return to play include signs of infection and suspicion of an embedded foreign body. In such cases, it is recommended that an ophthalmologist be consulted for further evaluation.

Consequences

Although often acutely painful, abrasion of the epithelial layer of the cornea heals very quickly (within days). However, an untreated corneal abrasion may predispose to severe infection, permanent scarring, and vision loss [18]. Additional trauma to the cornea, such as rubbing the eyes or introduction of another foreign body, may cause the area of injury to expand, thus delaying the healing process. Secondary complications, including corneal infection, may rarely complicate cases of corneal abrasion [19].

1.2.2.2 Eyelid Abrasion and Laceration

Facial and eyelid lacerations are among the most common basketball-related injuries. Uncomplicated lacerations to the body or face can be addressed courtside with primary closure [20]. Lacerations involving the upper and/or lower eyelid have the risk of impacting the canalicular system, which functions to drain tears from the eye, or the underlying levator palpebrae superioris muscle, which elevates and retracts the upper eyelid [5]. The mechanism of injury can be due to blunt (e.g., elbow or the basketball) or sharp (e.g., fingernail) trauma. Injuries to the eyelid can be categorized in three ways: eyelid laceration without marginal involvement, eyelid laceration with marginal involvement (Fig. 1.3), and eyelid laceration with canalicular system involvement (Fig. 1.4). More extensive injuries may involve all three categories.

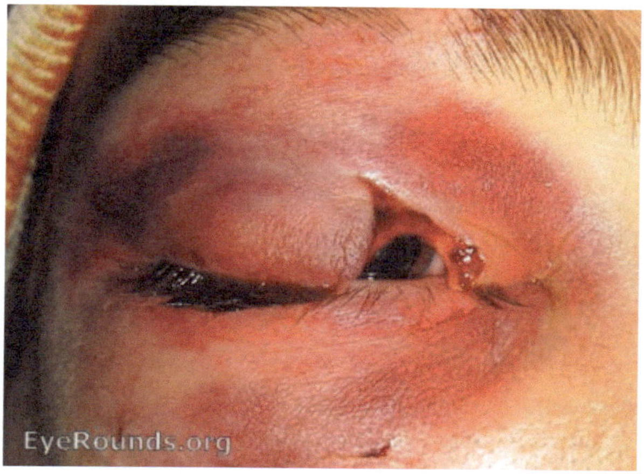

Fig. 1.3 A full thickness upper eyelid laceration with marginal involvement. (Source: Image from EyeRounds.org, The University of Iowa and reprinted with permission from Dr. Thomas A Oetting, MD (https://eyerounds.org/atlas/pages/lid-laceration-full-thickness.html#gsc.tab=0) under Creative Commons License (https://creativecommons.org/licenses/by-nc-nd/3.0/deed.en))

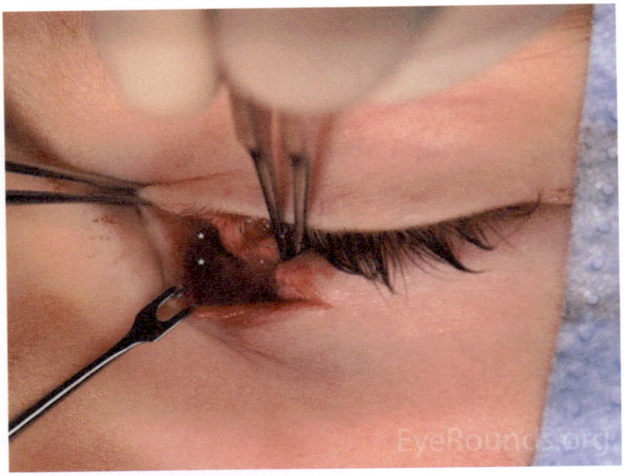

Fig. 1.4 A full thickness lower eyelid laceration with canalicular system involvement. The proximal lacerated end of the canaliculus (asterisk) is present deep within the medial canthus. (Source: Image from EyeRounds.org, The University of Iowa and reprinted with permission from Dr. Thomas A. Oetting, MD (https://webeye.ophth.uiowa.edu/eyeforum/atlas/pages/canalicular-lacerations.htm#gsc.tab=0) under Creative Commons License (https://creativecommons.org/licenses/by-nc-nd/3.0/deed.en))

Clinical Findings

Eyelid lacerations may present differently depending on the size and location of the laceration. They are typically associated with acute eye pain, bleeding and erythema, and edema of the surrounding tissue. Deep lacerations that result in injury to the underlying levator palpebrae superioris muscle may present with ptosis (eyelid drooping) and protrusion of orbital fat. Lacerations near the orbital rim may result in supra- or infraorbital anesthesia. Computed tomography (CT) of the head and/or orbit may be required in some cases to exclude other intracranial or periorbital injuries, especially if there is a history of loss of conscious or any suspicion for penetrating injury or severe blunt trauma [21]. Due to the complexity of the eyelids and the possibility of hidden underlying injuries, it is recommended that all eyelid lacerations undergo thorough examination by an ophthalmologist [22].

Treatment

An eyelid laceration without marginal involvement can often be closed primarily under local anesthesia in the locker room or in the clinic. Smaller lacerations can be closed courtside using topical skin adhesive, without the need for sutures. When the eyelid margin and/or the canalicular system are involved, the repair may need to be performed in the operating room with or without sedation and monitored anesthesia. A canalicular laceration may require an oculoplastic specialist to place an indwelling stent [13]. To minimize risk of infection, irrigation of the laceration and administration of an oral antibiotic regimen may be indicated. Prophylaxis for tetanus should also be considered depending on the patient's immunization status [21, 23].

Return to Play

Recommendations for returning to play in cases of eyelid lacerations are largely dependent on the size, location, and severity of the laceration. For small lacerations without marginal involvement, return to play may be indicated immediately after primary closure. However, in more severe cases or if an underlying globe injury is suspected, ample evaluation, treatment, and recovery time will be needed.

Consequences

Proper positioning and structure of the eyelids is important in protecting the globe, maintaining the tear film, and facilitating tear movement and drainage. An untreated or improperly treated eyelid laceration may result in a variety of complications associated with disruption of these functions.

1.2.2.3 Orbital Fracture

Around the eye, cranial bones articulate to form the orbit, a bony structure that protects the contents that lie within (globe, extraocular muscles, lacrimal apparatus, blood vessels, nerves, and adipose tissue). The orbit is separated structurally into four walls: the orbital roof, medial wall, lateral wall, and orbital floor [24]. A blowout fracture is a specific type of orbital fracture characterized by fracture of the orbital wall into an adjacent paranasal sinus. Because the orbital floor and medial wall are the thinnest orbital walls, most blowout fractures are a result of these bones buckling under the force of blunt trauma [25, 26]. A trapdoor fracture is another type of orbital fracture that is more common in children. Due to the soft texture of young bone, a fractured orbital wall (particularly with a small deficit) quickly rebounds to its original position, resulting in minimal radiographic evidence of a fracture. Often the eye appears quiet without obvious signs of trauma, but there may be marked entrapment of orbital contents within the fracture, leading to restricted extraocular motility or tissue ischemia [26, 27]. These fractures are often referred to as "white-eyed blowout fractures" and often require prompt attention [28].

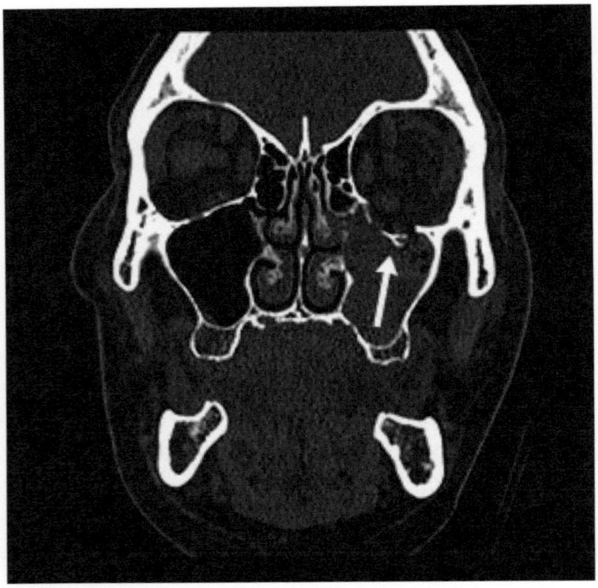

Fig. 1.5 A discontinuity in the inferior orbital wall of the left eye is seen on coronal orbital computed tomography (CT) scan (arrow). (Source: Image from the University of Michigan Kellogg Eye Center and reprinted with permission from Dr. Jonathan D. Trobe, MD (https://kellogg.umich.edu/theeyeshaveit/trauma/orbital_fracture.html) under Creative Commons Attribution 3.0 License)

Clinical Findings

Clinical findings of an orbital fracture largely depend on the location, extent, and type of fracture that has occurred. As a result, all patients with a suspected orbital fracture should undergo a complete ophthalmic examination, which includes assessment of visual acuity, ocular motility, intraocular pressure, and globe position. Some common findings include periorbital pain and ecchymosis, restriction of extraocular motility, decreased visual function, eyelid edema or bruising, subcutaneous emphysema, enophthalmos or hypoglobus, diplopia, and hypoesthesia in the supraorbital or infraorbital nerve distribution. Entrapment of an extraocular muscle may result in signs and symptoms of the oculobradycardiac reflex which include bradycardia, somnolence, lethargy, and nausea. Computed tomography (CT) of the orbit and midface is typically suggested for all patients with a suspected orbital fracture (Fig. 1.5) [21]. Depending on the extent of head trauma, patients who suffer from an orbital fracture may present with headache, loss of consciousness, nausea/vomiting, and dizziness [29].

Treatment

If there is clinical suspicion for extraocular muscle entrapment, such as a marked ductional deficit, persistent bradycardia, nausea or vomiting, or syncope, urgent surgical exploration and repair of the fracture should be performed. Surgical repair is indicated within 1–2 weeks for fractures with persistent diplopia, large orbital floor or combined medial wall and floor fractures, and complex fractures involving the orbital rim, lateral wall, or zygomatic arch [21]. Oral antibiotics should be considered for patients with coinciding sinusitis, diabetes mellitus, or those who are immunocompromised. Orbital edema can be addressed with the use of ice packs and/or oral corticosteroids. Local nasal decongestants are an option to reduce sinus pressure [13, 26].

Return to Play

Recommendations for returning to play will differ depending on the location and extent of the fracture itself as well as any additional injuries to the orbit or globe. Orbital strength and stability should be assessed based on clinical signs and ophthalmic examination findings. In most cases, athletes are able to return to play after about 3–6 weeks of wound healing [30].

Consequences

Patients who experience any fracture to the orbit should be monitored for any persistent diplopia, enophthalmos, or development of ocular injuries such as retinal detachment, orbital cellulitis, or angle-recession glaucoma. When evaluating the patient with orbital fracture, care must be taken to exclude any damage to the globe or optic nerve. Patients should be counseled to avoid nose blowing, which may introduce air into the orbital fracture site and create an orbital compartment syndrome resulting in optic nerve compression. Delay or failure to release any entrapped muscle may result in muscle ischemia and fibrosis, which may lead to permanent restrictive strabismus [21].

1.2.2.4 Traumatic Iritis

Iritis, also known as anterior uveitis, is inflammation of the vascular uveal layer of the eye, specifically at the iris. Iritis can be caused by blunt trauma to the eye, in which damage to the iris prompts an inflammatory response on the anterior chamber of the eye. This inflammatory response can lead to damage to the ciliary body, accumulation of debris in the trabecular meshwork, and damage to the iris sphincter (Fig. 1.6) [31].

Clinical Findings

Traumatic iritis typically presents as a dull, aching, or throbbing pain that develops within 1–3 days of trauma. Along with the pain, patients may experience eye redness, tearing, photophobia, and diminished vision. A slit lamp examination may show inflammatory white blood cells in the anterior chamber [13, 21]. There may

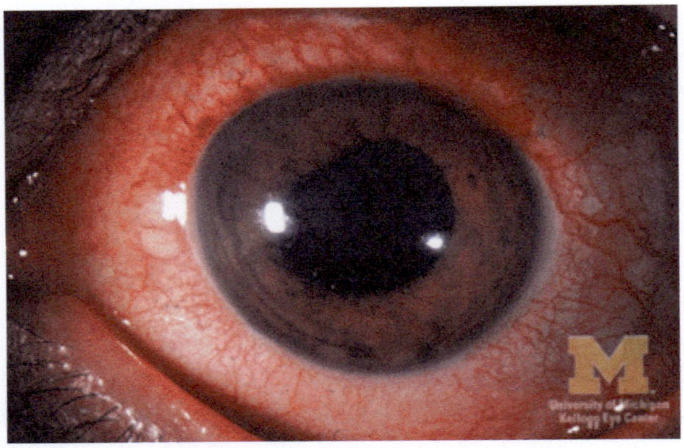

Fig. 1.6 Engorged conjunctival vessels (ciliary flush) and an irregularly shaped pupil in traumatic iritis. (Source: Image from the University of Michigan Kellogg Eye Center and reprinted with permission from Dr. Jonathan D. Trobe, MD (https://kellogg.umich.edu/theeyeshaveit/redeye/anterior_uveitis.html) under Creative Commons Attribution 3.0 License)

also be keratitic precipitates on the corneal endothelium or posterior iris synechiae. The intraocular pressure (IOP) of the affected eye may be different from the unaffected eye. A higher IOP would be due to accumulation of inflammatory debris in the trabecular meshwork, while a lower IOP may result from ciliary body damage [21].

Treatment

Pain with traumatic iritis can be managed with cycloplegic eye drops that immobilize the ciliary body, preventing muscle spasms that cause pain or discomfort. Inflammation can be addressed with topical steroids [21].

Return to Play

Symptoms usually improve within 1–2 days after initiation of steroid therapy, after which return to play is permitted.

Consequences

While most patients respond well to steroid therapy, there is a risk of recurrence or persistent symptoms. A full ocular exam should be conducted if there is suspicion of deeper damage, especially when the iritis is a result of perforating or penetrating injuries [31]. Some additional complications include decreased visual acuity, secondary glaucoma (due to angle recession or accumulation of inflammatory debris in the trabecular meshwork), retinal damage or detachment, cataract, and macular edema [21].

1.2.2.5 Globe Rupture

Penetrating and perforating globe injuries may occur from full-thickness injury to the cornea or sclera; however, they differ in their mechanisms of injury. A globe rupture is caused by blunt trauma which causes an acute increase in intraocular pressure (IOP). This results in an inside-out force that ruptures the eyewall at its weakest point and commonly results in tissue herniation. A globe laceration is caused by a sharp object penetrating (entry wound only) or perforating (entry and exit wounds) the eyewall [32]. Because a globe laceration results in immediate decompression of the globe, there may not be any acute elevation of IOP and secondary hypotony may occur. Immediate protection with minimal manipulation is recommended in such circumstances to prevent further injury at the site [33]. Of these two injuries, globe ruptures due to blunt trauma are far more common in basketball and thus will be the focus of this section.

Clinical Findings

Clinically, a globe rupture is the most severe form of an ocular injury due to damage and exposure of the intraocular contents. As such, any suspicion of a ruptured globe warrants immediate evaluation of the eye by an ophthalmologist. Evaluation of globe rupture should be done with minimal manipulation of the injured eye to prevent further damage. Diagnosis is commonly made clinically using slip lamp examination, indirect ophthalmoscopy/funduscopy, or a penlight [21]. A computed tomography (CT) scan may be indicated in cases where thorough visualization of the globe is not possible and may also be used to identify orbital fracture or intraocular pathologies (e.g., foreign bodies, lens dislocation, retinal detachment, or hemorrhage) [34].

Common locations of traumatic globe rupture are where the sclera is the weakest and thinnest, including the limbus (the area where the cornea and sclera meet) and posterior to the insertion of extraocular muscles [35]. Associated symptoms include eye pain, decreased visual acuity, loss of fluid leading to low IOP, and restriction of extraocular movements. The presence of subconjunctival hemorrhage, hyphema, or vitreous hemorrhage may obscure some damaged areas, so it is important to conduct a thorough ophthalmic examination which may need to take place under anesthesia. Structural deformities to the globe include shallowing or deepening of the anterior chamber, peaking or deforming of the pupil, iridodialysis (separation of the iris from the ciliary body), or cyclodialysis (separation of the ciliary muscle fibers from the scleral spur). Further examination may reveal lens material or vitreous fluid in the anterior chamber, intraocular tissue prolapse, and retinal damage [21, 34]. Another serious complication of an open globe injury is endophthalmitis [36].

Treatment

Treatment of globe rupture is surgical repair by an ophthalmologist as soon as possible, ideally within 24 h. The primary goals of repair are to restore the structural integrity of the globe wall and to avoid prolapse of any intraocular contents [37]. Once a diagnosis of globe rupture has been made, the affected eye should be protected with a hard shield at all times prior to surgical repair. To prevent infection, preoperative antibiotics should be administered no later than 6 h post injury. In cases with high risk of infection or endophthalmitis, such as prolonged delay until surgical repair, retained intraocular foreign bodies, and rupture of the lens capsule, intravitreal antibiotics may be administered during surgical repair. Additional pharmacologic treatment includes antiemetics to prevent any Valsalva maneuvers and subsequent expulsion of intraocular contents and tetanus toxoid booster if vaccination history is incomplete or uncertain. Pain medications are indicated pre- and post-operatively as needed [21].

Return to Play

Any suspicion or evidence of open globe precludes return to play and should be thoroughly investigated by an ophthalmologist. Strenuous physical activity or any Valsalva maneuvers before surgical repair may worsen prolapse of intraocular tissue. The recovery period after surgery is also prolonged to minimize any activity that may lead to re-rupture of the globe. Guidance regarding when a player is able to return to the court after a globe rupture requires assessment by an ophthalmologist [13].

Consequences

The prognosis of a globe rupture can be assessed using the Ocular Trauma Score (OTS), which considers variables such as the patient's initial presenting vision and the presence of any complications. Ocular tissue herniation and prolapse of intraocular contents are common complications of globe rupture due to the inside-out mechanism of trauma [21]. A notable sequela of iridodialysis is risk of angle recession and elevation of IOP, which may contribute to the development of traumatic glaucoma. Conversely, iridodialysis and/or cyclodialysis can result in an alternate pathway of drainage for aqueous humor and thus low IOP, or ocular hypotony [38]. Some additional complications of globe rupture include endophthalmitis, retinal detachment, and afferent pupillary defect [21]. As such, it is crucial to manage any open globe injury with broad-spectrum antibiotics and surgical repair as soon as possible.

1.2.2.6 Retinal Tear and Detachment

A retinal tear is an ocular injury in basketball where trauma to the globe causes a full-thickness break in the retina. This break can subsequently result in a rhegmatogenous retinal detachment, in which the vitreous fluid collects within the subretinal space, between the neurosensory retina and the retinal pigment epithelium (Fig. 1.7). Although less common among other basketball-related eye injuries, retinal tears and detachments are serious injuries that may require surgical repair [39].

Players with myopia are at higher risk of developing a retinal tear and subsequent retinal detachment upon blunt trauma to the eye, and this risk increases with the amount of myopia. As such, protective eyewear is recommended for basketball players with high myopia [40, 41].

Clinical Findings

The most common symptom of a retinal tear is the presence of flashes or floaters. Depending on the severity of the retinal tear, visual acuity may be affected. In cases of retinal detachment, players will experience vision loss. This is often described as a shadow or curtain moving over their field of vision and may be peripheral or central. A large retinal detachment may present with a relative afferent pupillary defect [21].

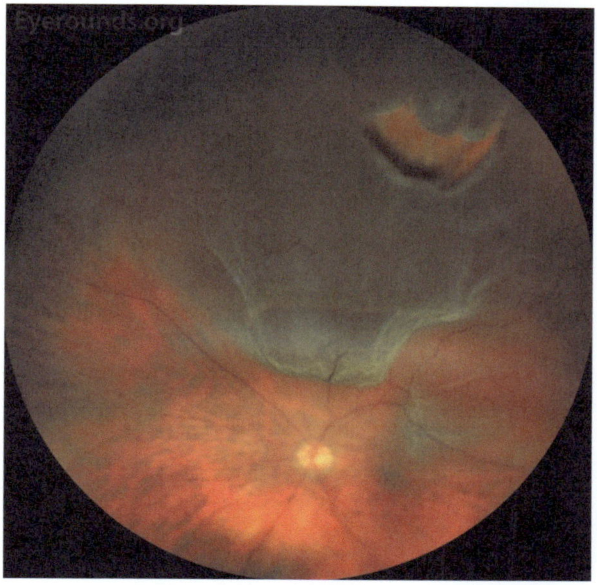

Fig. 1.7 A superior horseshoe retinal tear and secondary macula-involving rhegmatogenous retinal detachment. (Source: Image from EyeRounds.org, The University of Iowa and reprinted with permission from Dr. Thomas A. Oetting, MD (https://eyerounds.org/atlas/pages/rhegmatogenous-ret-detach.htm#gsc.tab=0) under Creative Commons License (https://creativecommons.org/licenses/by-nc-nd/3.0/deed.en))

Any suspicion of a retinal tear or subsequent retinal detachment should warrant urgent referral to an ophthalmologist. Diagnosis should first involve an anterior vitreous evaluation using a slit lamp to check for the presence of retinal pigment epithelial cells released from the tear (Shafer's sign). A trauma-induced rhegmatogenous retinal detachment has a corrugated and opaque appearance upon dilated indirect ophthalmoscopy/funduscopy, unlike the smooth appearances of tractional or serous retinal detachments. Other findings include posterior vitreous detachment, vitreous hemorrhage, the presence of subretinal fluid that does not shift with gravity, and an operculum (free-floating piece of the retina). If the retina is unable to be visualized due to opacities, ultrasound may be used to aid diagnosis [21].

Treatment

For acute retinal tears without evidence of detachment, transconjunctival cryopexy or laser photocoagulation should be performed within 24 h of the trauma [42]. This process secures the surrounding retina to the retinal pigment epithelial layer and may prevent a detachment. If detachment has already occurred, surgical repair is indicated. In cases where the detachment is near the macula, surgery should be done as soon as possible to prevent progression of the tear to involve the macula. Otherwise, the procedure can be performed within 7–10 days of the trauma [21]. Additional measures can be done to support the eye, including removal of vitreous fluid to limit traction on the retina, use of a silicone scleral buckle to provide mechanical support to the globe, and placement of a gas bubble to tamponade the retina to the retinal pigment epithelium [13].

Return to Play

Any suspicion or evidence of retinal tear or detachment should be thoroughly investigated by an ophthalmologist and return to play is not permitted until the lesion is repaired. Retinal tears without detachment have a shorter duration of recovery and players may return to play days to weeks after receiving laser treatment or cryotherapy. Cases of retinal detachment warrant longer recovery times of weeks to months before players should return to play [13]. In either situation, players should follow-up with an ophthalmologist after treatment to determine if return to play is indicated [21].

Consequences

Following retinal repair, intraretinal fibrosis and proliferative membranes may form on the inner and outer surfaces of the retina and vitreous. These membranes generally consist of retinal pigment epithelial and glial cells that grow and contract, also known as proliferative vitreoretinopathy [43]. In addition to a poor visual outcome due to retinal dysfunction, some further consequences of this complication include irregularities in the retinal pigment epithelium, puckering of the macula, cystoid macular edema, and subretinal fibrosis [44].

1.2.2.7 Subconjunctival Hemorrhage

A subconjunctival hemorrhage occurs when conjunctival or episcleral blood vessels rupture and leak blood between the conjunctiva and the sclera, also known as the subconjunctival space. The conjunctiva is the clear layer of surface epithelial tissue, and the sclera is the rigid layer of white connective tissue that is continuous with the cornea and provides structural integrity and protection to the eye [11]. Bleeding into the subconjunctival space can be caused by an impact trauma to the site of hemorrhage (e.g., another player or the basketball hitting the eye), after Valsalva maneuver (e.g., forceful coughing, sneezing, or blowing the nose), or even after minor trauma that the patient does not recall (e.g., rubbing the eye) [45].

Clinical Findings

A case of subconjunctival hemorrhage typically presents acutely as a sharply demarcated region of extravasated blood without any impact on vision (Fig. 1.8). Large collections of blood that elevate the conjunctiva may cause mild irritation and the feeling of a foreign body [13]. While many cases of subconjunctival hemorrhage have only minor consequences, all traumatic cases should undergo a thorough eye examination to exclude other ocular injuries such as a ruptured globe or conjunctival laceration [45].

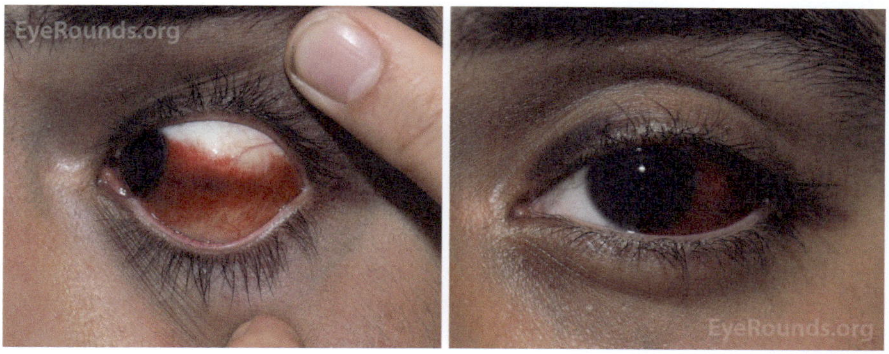

Fig. 1.8 Blood accumulation between the conjunctiva and sclera in a traumatic subconjunctival hemorrhage. (Source: Image from EyeRounds.org, The University of Iowa and reprinted with permission from Dr. Thomas A. Oetting, MD (https://webeye.ophth.uiowa.edu/eyeforum/atlas/pages/Subconjunctival-Hemorrhage.html#gsc.tab=0) under Creative Commons License (https://creativecommons.org/licenses/by-nc-nd/3.0/deed.en))

Treatment

There is generally no treatment indicated for a subconjunctival hemorrhage. Within a few weeks, the extravasated blood will be reabsorbed and the contusion will resolve on its own. If there is a large collection of blood that elevates the conjunctiva and causes some irritation, application of artificial tears or ointment can lubricate the eye and improve comfort [13]. A cold compress can also be used to provide further comfort and reduce tissue swelling.

Return to Play

Because the risk of vision loss is minimal, there is no contraindication to immediately returning to play after an isolated subconjunctival hemorrhage. There is, however, an exception to be made for extensive subconjunctival hemorrhage where the blood collection extends to large areas around the eye. In such cases, return to play should be delayed until the eye can be examined by an ophthalmologist for a more occult ocular injury (e.g., scleral rupture or open globe injury) [13].

Consequences

Subconjunctival hemorrhage alone typically has a good prognosis with spontaneous resolution. With minimal eye discomfort and visual impact, there are no significant consequences associated with an isolated subconjunctival hemorrhage. However, it is important to note that persistent or recurrent episodes of subconjunctival hemorrhage may be indicative of more dangerous underlying conditions such as coagulopathies or more extensive concomitant pathology such as an orbital fracture or retinal detachment [46].

1.2.2.8 Traumatic Hyphema

A traumatic hyphema occurs when blunt trauma causes shearing of the microvasculature in the anterior chamber of the eye. Another mechanism of injury is a contusive trauma that causes a rapid increase in intraocular pressure (IOP) that ruptures the microvasculature. As a result of these injuries, clotted or unclotted blood pools within the anterior chamber, either partially or completely filling the chamber between the cornea and the iris (Fig. 1.9) [47]. The blood may appear as red (oxygenated) or black (deoxygenated) in the chamber, and the hyphema may be visible without a slit lamp [21].

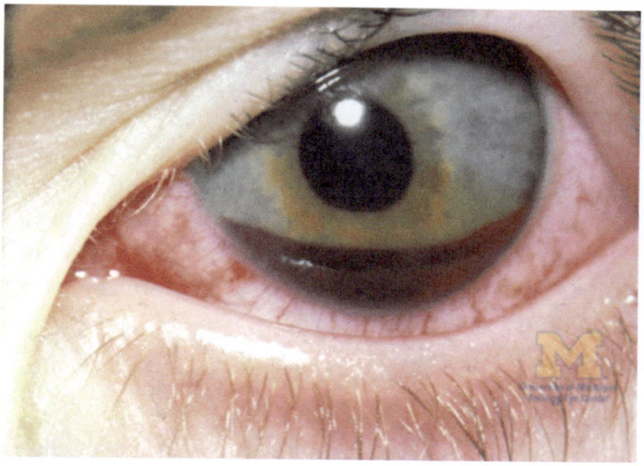

Fig. 1.9 Blood accumulation in the anterior chamber of the eye in a traumatic hyphema. (Source: Image from the University of Michigan Kellogg Eye Center and reprinted with permission from Dr. Jonathan D. Trobe, MD (https://kellogg.umich.edu/theeyeshaveit/trauma/hyphema.html) under Creative Commons Attribution 3.0 License)

Clinical Findings

Traumatic hyphema is generally a self-limiting condition with symptoms of eye pain and a sudden decrease in visual acuity or loss of vision in the affected eye [21]. Severe complications, particularly with more extensive bleeding that may cause permanent damage to the eye, include corneal staining, elevated IOP, secondary inflammation, and secondary hemorrhage (rebleeding). These will be further discussed in the "Consequences" section.

Assessment of a traumatic hyphema should include a thorough ocular examination to inspect for any additional injuries to the eye such as globe rupture, retinal detachment, or orbital fracture. The use of ultrasound and computed tomography (CT) is indicated if the hyphema interferes with evaluation of such injuries. The extent, height, and location of the hyphema should be assessed using slit lamp biomicroscopy. IOP should be measured daily via tonometry to identify any development of glaucoma. It is important to note, however, that diagnostic methods that deform the globe (e.g., scleral depression or gonioscopy) should generally be avoided to limit the risk of rebleed [21, 47, 48].

Treatment

Most cases of traumatic hyphema are self-limited and can clear without any surgical intervention. Supportive care should be centered around limiting activity to avoid a rebleed and elevation of the head to allow the blood to settle. A protective shield of rigid plastic or metal should be placed over the affected eye as it heals, particularly within the first 10 days after initial trauma [13]. However, it is important to avoid patching the eye, as this would prevent timely identification of a rebleed. Mild analgesics such as acetaminophen can be given for symptom control, while aspirin and anticoagulants are generally avoided. Topical steroids are indicated in the case of any secondary inflammation; however, it is important to taper the steroids as soon as inflammatory signs resolve to prevent development of glaucoma. Topical cycloplegics should be given to prevent movement of the ciliary muscle which may enlarge the hyphema [21].

Patients with non-clearing hyphemas (blood does not clear by 50% in 8 days), those with secondary glaucoma, or significant decrease in vision should be considered for surgical evacuation of the hyphema. Patients with increased risk of rebleeding, such as those with systemic blood disorders (including sickle-cell disease), larger hyphemas, delayed evaluation, and use of antiplatelet or anticoagulant medications, may require more aggressive treatment with the potential for hospitalization [47, 48].

Return to Play

Return to play should be delayed until the hyphema is resolved. It is commonly recommended that athletes should wait at least 1 week after initial trauma before participating in any strenuous physical activities, even if the hyphema is no longer visible. Athletes should continue to wear protective eyewear for at least 1 month to limit risk of secondary hemorrhage [13, 21].

Consequences

Traumatic hyphema is often self-limited. However, there are a number of potential complications that may result in a poor ocular outcome.

The deposition of erythrocytes, fibrin, platelets, and other debris in the trabecular meshwork (spongy tissue that drains aqueous humor) can cause a buildup of aqueous humor and elevated IOP. This manifests as acute eye pain and may lead to secondary angle-recession glaucoma and permanent damage to the optic nerve. Late glaucoma can also develop weeks to years after the initial trauma, caused by secondary hemorrhage due to rebleeding angle recession [13, 47].

As blood pools in the anterior chamber, erythrocytes stain the interior surface of the cornea and can lead to corneal opacification and loss of vision. The risk of corneal staining is particularly high in large hyphemas with prolonged clot retraction, corneal epithelial damage, and persistently high IOP [47]. There is also concern for the development of secondary intraocular inflammation, iritis, and peripheral anterior synechiae (adhesions between adjacent structures) due to blood collection within the anterior chamber [13, 48].

Another common finding is the development of secondary hemorrhage (rebleeding) into the anterior chamber due to clot lysis and retraction. These bleeds are generally worse than the initial hyphema and patients are thus more at risk of developing the previously described complications. Patients with sickle-cell trait and other systemic blood dyscrasia may be at risk of secondary hemorrhage and therefore require more aggressive initial treatment. Increased risk of rebleeding is also associated with delayed evaluation of the initial trauma, larger hyphema size, worse initial visual acuity, and the use of antiplatelet medications [47].

1.2.2.9 Commotio Retinae

Commotio retinae is a type of traumatic retinopathy that is described as confluent whitening of the periphery or posterior pole (Berlin edema) of the retina. This whitening reflects damage due to shearing of the photoreceptors as a result of shock waves from the traumatic impact. Specifically, fragmentation of the outer segments of photoreceptors leads to depigmentation as well as extra- and intracellular edema. Depending on the circumstances of the trauma, the impacted area can appear at the site of impact (coup) or at distant sites (contrecoup).

Clinical Findings

Clinical presentation of commotio retinae varies depending on the extent of retinal involvement and the presence of other ocular injuries. When commotio retinae occurs in the periphery, patients are often asymptomatic. When retinal whitening occurs closer to the macula, patients may experience a decrease in visual acuity; severe trauma may cause injury to the inner retinal layers and result in permanent vision loss. It is important to note, however, that the degree of visual impairment is not necessarily reflected by the degree of retinal whitening. Depending on the severity of trauma, additional ocular injuries such as retinal hemorrhage or retinal detachment may be present [21].

Assessment of suspected commotio retinae involves a thorough ophthalmic examination. Dilated ophthalmoscopy/funduscopy should be done to visualize the area of retinal whitening and retinal blood vessels that remain undisturbed. Intraretinal hemorrhages and retinal pigment epithelium mottling may be observed. Peripheral retinal examination should be conducted with scleral depression in cases where globe rupture, hyphema, and iritis are excluded [21, 49].

Treatment

Commotio retinae is a self-limited condition that does not require any treatment. The visual deficit typically improves with a good visual outcome in most patients. Care should be taken to reassess the patient 1–2 weeks after the initial injury for any concomitant injury to the posterior globe such as a retinal detachment or a choroidal rupture. Patients should be educated to return for prompt evaluation should any new visual symptoms occur [21].

Return to Play

Due to the mild nature of the injury, players are able to return to play after evaluation via dilated eye examination and consultation with an ophthalmologist [13].

Consequences

Although the clinical findings of commotio retinae are mild, it is important to consider the possibility of a more serious ocular injury as a result of the initial trauma. Retinal tear, detachment, and injury to the choroid may have been overlooked upon initial evaluation and should be thoroughly excluded before a diagnosis of isolated commotio retinae is made.

1.2.3 Eye Protection in Basketball

In 2004, the American Academy of Pediatrics and the American Academy of Ophthalmology formed the Eye Health and Public Information Task Force. In a joint policy statement, they strongly recommended the use of protective eyewear for basketball players of all ages and skill ranges. This task force further recommended that mandatory protective eyewear should be worn by athletes who are functionally monocular and those who have experienced eye trauma and/or surgery in the past [50]. Despite these recommendations, over 95% of professional players who experienced basketball-related ocular injuries did not wear eye protection while playing, and there are currently no requirements or standards by sports governing bodies for protective eyewear in the United States [20].

Eye protection should ideally have lenses made from impact-resistant polycarbonate or Trivex, which are able to disperse the force of impact and thus prevent ocular injury [51]. It is important to note that contact lenses and standard prescription glasses offer little protection and are not substitutes for protective eyewear. Individuals who require refractive lens prescriptions should wear a polycarbonate lens with the prescription included, contact lenses plus non-prescriptive eye protection, or eye protection that is able to be worn over standard prescription glasses [50].

The literature surrounding the epidemiology of eye trauma in basketball is limited, and the use of eye protection during play remains unpopular. Increased attention to the prevalence of eye trauma in basketball, as well as the benefits of eye protection in basketball, is crucial in promoting the use of protective measures to prevent injury. Additionally, eye protection is particularly important after an ocular injury to prevent worsening of an existing deficit [52]. Ophthalmologists are encouraged to prevent basketball-related eye injuries through patient education and awareness.

1.3 Visual Performance in Basketball

1.3.1 Visual Training for Athletes

Although a very physical sport, the dynamic nature of basketball requires players to be aware of a variety of positional and temporal factors related to the ball, players, and the hoop. Some visual functions identified as critical to the success of players in basketball are visual acuity, oculomotor coordination, accommodation, stereopsis (visuospatial perception), and visual information processing [53, 54]. Players who have a greater ability to process visual input quickly and execute the appropriate motor actions have been thought to have an advantage. As such, basketball players may undergo visual performance training to improve visual function and performance outcomes. Analysis of vision is often done using Eye Tracking Glasses (ETG) to understand the dynamics of visuomotor tasks and assess how various parameters can relate to basketball performance [55].

1.3.1.1 Visual Tracking Speed

There is a lack of scientific consensus on the correlation of visual-motor reaction speed with athletic performance in basketball. It is proposed that perceptual-cognitive capability and visual tracking speed (VTS) are better explanations for the ability of superior athletes to produce a more effective performance. A player's VTS is the speed at which multiple objects are tracked visually [56].

Being able to efficiently devote cognitive resources toward the processing of visual information allows players to reach a motor decision more rapidly, which translates to a higher VTS [57]. One study involving players in the National Basketball Association (NBA) found a relationship between the number of positive plays and a player's VTS. It was proposed that a higher VTS relates to a greater ability of the player to see and respond to multiple stimuli at one time. As a result, those players are able to keep track of and respond to a variety of ongoing actions in a timely manner [56]. Visual tracking speed can be improved through reactive agility training involving a diversity of exercises that require the player to constantly and rapidly change the direction and location of their movements [58].

1.3.1.2 Visual Gaze Control

Quiet eye is a term used to describe the act of tracking a specific location or object for at least 100 ms. This period of quiet eye is thought to correspond with the preparatory time it takes players to organize neural networks that are needed to prepare for movement control [59]. During high pressure situations, athletes experience anxiety and heightened emotions, causing attention shifts and shorter quiet eye periods which negatively impact performance. This is especially important for basketball players in their ability to execute far-aiming tasks, such as a free throw and three-point shot [60].

It has been shown that longer periods of quiet eye correlate with positive performance measures such as increased accuracy of shots. Furthermore, quiet eye duration is trainable. A study involving elite and novice basketball players demonstrated that training to extend the duration of quiet eye had improved basketball performance when compared with a control group [61]. This phenomenon is further supported by a similar investigation within the context of golf putting. Golfers who were trained to have longer quiet eye periods exhibited expedited learning and resistance to anxiety during performance when compared to players who received only technical training [62].

1.3.2 Visuomotor Benefits of Basketball

A number of studies support the idea that athletes tend to present with better visual function than individuals with no sporting background. There has been some debate in the past related to whether these differences are related to innate abilities of an athlete that allows them to be successful in the sport or whether these abilities are developed and improved through practice and training. There are also questions regarding the extent to which successful athletes benefit from superior visual skills or if perceptual and cognitive skills hold a greater weight [53, 63].

Thus far, consensus supports the position that discrepancies found between athletes and sedentary individuals are largely due to constant practice and training programs, and that innate contributions are not as important [54, 64, 65]. It is important, however, to remain aware of innate differences between an athlete's baseline visual ability, as well as perceptual and cognitive skill, which may impact the performance on the court. As such, there is increased support for a multidimensional explanation behind athlete performance as it relates to visuomotor skill.

Many nuances and mechanisms behind the visuomotor benefits of basketball are still being studied and thus are not well delineated [63]. Despite the lack of solid conclusions to date, we are able to draw preliminary connections between participation in dynamic sports such as basketball and the improvement of visual performance skills over time. Increased attention into this field may help explain the mechanisms behind visual performance and visual information processing. A greater understanding may also allow visual training techniques to serve as a potential method of improving function for individuals with impaired vision [54].

1.4 Summary

Basketball is a common sport to produce ocular and orbital injuries. Clinicians should be aware of the ophthalmic aspects of basketball injuries in both recreational and professional players. Early recognition and treatment may be vision saving in many cases and may allow rehabilitation and return to play. Some ocular injuries (e.g., globe rupture, eyelid laceration, traumatic iritis, hyphema, or retinal detachment) may require urgent ophthalmic assessment, treatment, and/or hospitalization. Techniques for visual performance enhancement remain an emerging area of study that suggests the need for additional research.

References

1. Toldi JP, Thomas JL. Evaluation and management of sports-related eye injuries. Curr Sports Med Rep. 2020;19(1):29. https://doi.org/10.1249/JSR.0000000000000677.
2. Larrison WI, Hersh PS, Kunzweiler T, Shingleton BJ. Sports-related ocular trauma. Ophthalmology. 1990;97(10):1265–9. https://doi.org/10.1016/S0161-6420(90)32421-1.
3. Haring RS, Sheffield ID, Canner JK, Schneider EB. Epidemiology of sports-related eye injuries in the United States. JAMA Ophthalmol. 2016;134(12):1382–90. https://doi.org/10.1001/jamaophthalmol.2016.4253.
4. Padegimas EM, Stepan JG, Stoker GE, Polites GM, Brophy RH. Epidemiology and severity of sports and recreation injuries presenting to a tertiary adult emergency department. Phys Sportsmed. 2016;44(3):263–8. https://doi.org/10.1080/00913847.2016.1171683.
5. Heimmel MR, Murphy MA. Ocular injuries in basketball and baseball: what are the risks and how can we prevent them? Curr Sports Med Rep. 2008;7(5):284. https://doi.org/10.1249/JSR.0b013e318186ffc5.
6. Kim EJ, Ganga A, Rana VK, Greenberg PB. The epidemiology of basketball-associated eye injuries in the United States, 2012–2021. Graefes Arch Clin Exp Ophthalmol. 2023;261(12):3675–8. https://doi.org/10.1007/s00417-023-06136-8.
7. Youn J, Sallis RE, Smith G, Jones K. Ocular injury rates in college sports. Med Sci Sports Exerc. 2008;40(3):428. https://doi.org/10.1249/MSS.0b013e31815e7263.
8. Boden BP, Pierpoint LA, Boden RG, Comstock RD, Kerr ZY. Eye injuries in high school and collegiate athletes. Sports Health. 2017;9(5):444–9. https://doi.org/10.1177/1941738117712425.
9. Go JA, Lin SY, Williams KJ, et al. Eye injuries in the National Basketball Association. Ophthalmology. 2020;127(5):696–7. https://doi.org/10.1016/j.ophtha.2019.12.016.
10. Karlson TA, Klein BEK. The incidence of acute hospital-treated eye injuries. Arch Ophthalmol. 1986;104(10):1473–6. https://doi.org/10.1001/archopht.1986.01050220067028.
11. Armstrong RA, Cubbidge RP. The eye and vision: an overview. In: Preedy VR, editor. Handbook of nutrition, diet and the eye. Academic Press; 2014. p. 3–9. https://doi.org/10.1016/B978-0-12-401717-7.00001-0.
12. Sliwicki AL, Orringer K. Corneal abrasions. Pediatr Rev. 2023;44(6):343–5. https://doi.org/10.1542/pir.2022-005537.
13. Wisely CE, Kim T. Ophthalmic trauma in basketball. In: Laver L, Kocaoglu B, Cole B, Arundale AJH, Bytomski J, Amendola A, editors. Basketball sports medicine and science. Springer; 2020. p. 239–49. https://doi.org/10.1007/978-3-662-61070-1_22.
14. Wipperman JL, Dorsch JN. Evaluation and management of corneal abrasions. Am Fam Physician. 2013;87(2):114–20.
15. Wilson SA, Last A. Management of corneal abrasions. Am Fam Physician. 2004;70(1):123–8.

16. Beyer H, Cherkas D. Corneal foreign body removal using a bent needle tip. Am J Emerg Med. 2012;30(3):489–90. https://doi.org/10.1016/j.ajem.2010.12.038.
17. Moreira LB, Kasetsuwan N, Sanchez D, Shah SS, LaBree L, McDonnell PJ. Toxicity of topical anesthetic agents to human keratocytes in vivo. J Cataract Refract Surg. 1999;25(7):975. https://doi.org/10.1016/S0886-3350(99)00075-9.
18. Saccomano SJ, Ferrara LR. Managing corneal abrasions in primary care. Nurse Pract. 2014;39(9):1. https://doi.org/10.1097/01.NPR.0000452977.99676.cf.
19. Guier CP, Stokkermans TJ. Corneal foreign body removal. In: StatPearls. StatPearls Publishing; 2024. Accessed 31 Mar 2024. http://www.ncbi.nlm.nih.gov/books/NBK554478/.
20. Zagelbaum BM. The National Basketball Association eye injury study. Arch Ophthalmol. 1995;113(6):749. https://doi.org/10.1001/archopht.1995.01100060075035.
21. Bagheri N, Wajda B, Calvo C, Durrani A. The Wills eye manual: office and emergency room diagnosis and treatment of eye disease. 8th ed. Wolters Kluwer; 2021.
22. Hatton MP, Thakker MM, Ray S. Orbital and adnexal trauma associated with open-globe injuries. Ophthalmic Plast Reconstr Surg. 2002;18(6):458.
23. Chiang E, Bee C, Harris GJ, Wells TS. Does delayed repair of eyelid lacerations compromise outcome? Am J Emerg Med. 2017;35(11):1766–7. https://doi.org/10.1016/j.ajem.2017.04.062.
24. Gospe SMI, Bhatti MT. Orbital anatomy. Int Ophthalmol Clin. 2018;58(2):5. https://doi.org/10.1097/IIO.0000000000000214.
25. Blowout Fracture – American Association for Pediatric Ophthalmology and Strabismus. Accessed 3 May 2024. https://aapos.org/glossary/blowout-fracture.
26. Joseph JM, Glavas IP. Orbital fractures: a review. Clin Ophthalmol. 2011;5:95–100. https://doi.org/10.2147/OPTH.S14972.
27. Phan LT, Jordan Piluek W, McCulley TJ. Orbital trapdoor fractures. Saudi J Ophthalmol. 2012;26(3):277–82. https://doi.org/10.1016/j.sjopt.2012.05.008.
28. Jordan DR, Allen LH, White J, Harvey J, Pashby R, Esmaeli B. Intervention within days for some orbital floor fractures: the white-eyed blowout. Ophthalmic Plast Reconstr Surg. 1998;14(6):379–90. https://doi.org/10.1097/00002341-199811000-00001.
29. Koenen L, Waseem M. Orbital floor fracture. In: StatPearls. StatPearls Publishing; 2023. Accessed 3 May 2024. http://www.ncbi.nlm.nih.gov/books/NBK534825/.
30. Gilliland GD, Gilliland G, Fincher T, et al. Timing of return to normal activities after orbital floor fracture repair. Plast Reconstr Surg. 2007;120(1):245. https://doi.org/10.1097/01.prs.0000264391.45642.08.
31. Logothetis HD, Leikin SM, Patrianakos T. Management of anterior segment trauma. Dis Mon. 2014;60(6):247–53. https://doi.org/10.1016/j.disamonth.2014.03.004.
32. Kuhn F, Morris R, Witherspoon CD, Heimann K, Jeffers JB, Treister G. A standardized classification of ocular trauma. Graefes Arch Clin Exp Ophthalmol. 1996;234(6):399–403. https://doi.org/10.1007/BF00190717.
33. Fabian ID, Eliashiv S, Moisseiev J, Tryfonides C, Alhalel A. Prognostic factors and visual outcomes of ruptured and lacerated globe injuries. Eur J Ophthalmol. 2014;24(2):273–8. https://doi.org/10.5301/ejo.5000364.
34. Chronopoulos A, Ong JM, Thumann G, Schutz JS. Occult globe rupture: diagnostic and treatment challenge. Surv Ophthalmol. 2018;63(5):694–9. https://doi.org/10.1016/j.survophthal.2018.04.001.
35. Bi H, Cui Y, Li Y, Wang X, Zhang J. Clinical characteristics and surgical problems of ruptured globe injury. Curr Ther Res Clin Exp. 2013;74:16–21. https://doi.org/10.1016/j.curtheres.2012.10.002.
36. Zhang Y, Zhang MN, Jiang CH, Yao Y, Zhang K. Endophthalmitis following open globe injury. Br J Ophthalmol. 2010;94(1):111–4. https://doi.org/10.1136/bjo.2009.164913.
37. Bhattacharjee H, Barman M, Bhattacharjee K. Globe rupture. In: Mukherjee B, Yuen H, editors. Emergencies of the Orbit and Adnexa. Springer India; 2017. p. 9–17. https://doi.org/10.1007/978-81-322-1807-4_3.

38. González-Martín-Moro J, Contreras-Martín I, Muñoz-Negrete FJ, Gómez-Sanz F, Zarallo-Gallardo J. Cyclodialysis: an update. Int Ophthalmol. 2017;37(2):441–57. https://doi.org/10.1007/s10792-016-0282-8.
39. Ghazi NG, Green WR. Pathology and pathogenesis of retinal detachment. Eye. 2002;16(4):411–21. https://doi.org/10.1038/sj.eye.6700197.
40. Lee TH, Chen YH, Kuo HK, et al. Retinal detachment associated with basketball-related eye trauma. Am J Ophthalmol. 2017;180:97–101. https://doi.org/10.1016/j.ajo.2017.05.025.
41. Wilkinson CP. Retinal detachment. In: Spaide RF, Ohno-Matsui K, Yannuzzi LA, editors. Pathologic myopia. Springer International Publishing; 2021. p. 347–56. https://doi.org/10.1007/978-3-030-74334-5_23.
42. Robinson RT, Wadsworth LT, Feman SS. Traumatic retinal tear in a basketball player. Curr Sports Med Rep. 2011;10(3):129. https://doi.org/10.1249/JSR.0b013e31821b8c16.
43. Idrees S, Sridhar J, Kuriyan AE. Proliferative vitreoretinopathy: a review. Int Ophthalmol Clin. 2019;59(1):221–40. https://doi.org/10.1097/IIO.0000000000000258.
44. Kiss CG, Richter-Müksch S, Sacu S, Benesch T, Velikay-Parel M. Anatomy and function of the macula after surgery for retinal detachment complicated by proliferative vitreoretinopathy. Am J Ophthalmol. 2007;144(6):872–877.e1. https://doi.org/10.1016/j.ajo.2007.08.001.
45. Tarlan B, Kiratli H. Subconjunctival hemorrhage: risk factors and potential indicators. Clin Ophthalmol. 2013;7:1163–70. https://doi.org/10.2147/OPTH.S35062.
46. Dhillon J, Nassrallah G, Nithianandan H, et al. Significance of subconjunctival hemorrhage in predicting ocular pathology for patients with orbital fracture. Can J Ophthalmol. 2023;58(4):295–301. https://doi.org/10.1016/j.jcjo.2022.02.003.
47. Brandt MT, Haug RH. Traumatic hyphema: a comprehensive review. J Oral Maxillofac Surg. 2001;59(12):1462–70. https://doi.org/10.1053/joms.2001.28284.
48. Gharaibeh A, Savage HI, Scherer RW, Goldberg MF, Lindsley K. Medical interventions for traumatic hyphema. Cochrane Database Syst Rev. 2019;2019(1):CD005431. https://doi.org/10.1002/14651858.CD005431.pub4.
49. Mansour AM, Green WR, Hogge C. Histopathology of commotio retinae. Retina. 1992;12(1):24.
50. American Academy of Pediatrics, Committee on Sports Medicine and Fitness, American Academy of Ophthalmology, Eye Health and Public Information Task Force. Protective eyewear for young athletes. Ophthalmology. 2004;111(3):600–3. https://doi.org/10.1016/j.ophtha.2003.12.027.
51. Filipe JAC, Rocha-Sousa A, Falcão-Reis F, Castro-Correia J. Modern sports eye injuries. Br J Ophthalmol. 2003;87(11):1336–9. https://doi.org/10.1136/bjo.87.11.1336.
52. Kim EJ, Ganga A, Rana VK, Greenberg PB. Basketball-associated eye injuries: a systematic review. R I Med J. 2023;106(2):40–2.
53. Quintana MS, Román IR, Calvo AL, Molinuevo JS. Perceptual visual skills in young highly skilled basketball players. Percept Mot Skills. 2007;104(2):547–61. https://doi.org/10.2466/pms.104.2.547-561.
54. Vera J, Jiménez R, Cárdenas D, Redondo B, García JA. Visual function, performance, and processing of basketball players vs. sedentary individuals. J Sport Health Sci. 2020;9(6):587–94. https://doi.org/10.1016/j.jshs.2017.05.001.
55. Marques R, Martins FML, Mendes R, Dias G. The use of eye tracking glasses in basketball shooting: a systematic review. J Phys Educ Sport. 2018;18(1):175–83. https://doi.org/10.7752/jpes.2018.01023.
56. Mangine GT, Hoffman JR, Wells AJ, et al. Visual tracking speed is related to basketball-specific measures of performance in NBA players. J Strength Cond Res. 2014;28(9):2406. https://doi.org/10.1519/JSC.0000000000000550.
57. Faubert J, Sidebottom L. Perceptual-cognitive training of athletes. J Clin Sport Psychol. 2012;6(1):85–102. https://doi.org/10.1123/jcsp.6.1.85.

58. Hassan AK, Alhumaid MM, Hamad BE. The effect of using reactive agility exercises with the FITLIGHT training system on the speed of visual reaction time and dribbling skill of basketball players. Sports. 2022;10(11):176. https://doi.org/10.3390/sports10110176.
59. Mann DTY, Coombes SA, Mousseau MB, Janelle CM. Quiet eye and the Bereitschaftspotential: visuomotor mechanisms of expert motor performance. Cogn Process. 2011;12(3):223–34. https://doi.org/10.1007/s10339-011-0398-8.
60. Moeinirad S, Abdoli B, Farsi A, Ahmadi N. Training visual attention improves basketball three-point shot performance under pressure. Sport Sci Health. 2022;18(3):853–61. https://doi.org/10.1007/s11332-021-00866-0.
61. Vine SJ, Wilson MR. The influence of quiet eye training and pressure on attention and visuomotor control. Acta Psychol. 2011;136(3):340–6. https://doi.org/10.1016/j.actpsy.2010.12.008.
62. Moore LJ, Vine SJ, Cooke A, Ring C, Wilson MR. Quiet eye training expedites motor learning and aids performance under heightened anxiety: the roles of response programming and external attention. Psychophysiology. 2012;49(7):1005–15. https://doi.org/10.1111/j.1469-8986.2012.01379.x.
63. Ryu D, Abernethy B, Mann DL, Poolton JM, Gorman AD. The role of central and peripheral vision in expert decision making. Perception. 2013;42(6):591–691. https://doi.org/10.1068/p7487.
64. Schwab S, Memmert D. The impact of a sports vision training program in youth field hockey players. J Sports Sci Med. 2012;11(4):624–31.
65. Quevedo-Junyent L, Aznar-Casanova JA, Merindano-Encina D, Cardona G, Solé-Fortó J. Comparison of dynamic visual acuity between water polo players and sedentary students. Res Q Exerc Sport. 2011;82(4):644–51. https://doi.org/10.1080/02701367.2011.10599801.

Chapter 2
Ophthalmology of Swimming and Water Polo

Tuan Nguyen, Chris Alabiad, and Andrew G. Lee

2.1 Introduction

Swimming involves a participant propelling themselves through water using specific types of stroke technique (e.g., freestyle, breaststroke, backstroke, and butterfly). Competitive swimming often takes place in varying distances, ranging from 50 meter, which entails explosive power and lightning-fast finishes, to 10 km, which involves endurance and strategic pacing. In these events, swimmers compete to achieve the fastest times and outperform their opponents [1].

Water polo, on the other hand, combines team sports and swimming: two teams of seven players aim to outscore their opponents via throwing a ball into each opposing team's goal. Water polo demands immense physiological stress with players demonstrating intense bursts of physical activity followed by intervals of lower physical intensity [2].

Author, Andrew G. Lee, MD, discloses that he has served or is serving as a consultant for the following companies: AstraZeneca, Alexion, Bristol Mayers Squibb, National Football League, Catalyst, Viridian, Ethyreal, NASA, US Department of Justice, Dompe, and Stoke.

T. Nguyen (✉)
Weill Cornell/Rockefeller/Sloan-Kettering Tri-Institutional MD-PhD Program,
New York, NY, USA
e-mail: Tun2001@med.cornell.edu

C. Alabiad
Department of Ophthalmology, Bascom Palmer Eye Institute,
University of Miami Miller School of Medicine, Miami, FL, USA

A. G. Lee
Department of Ophthalmology, Blanton Eye Institute, Houston Methodist Hospital,
Houston, TX, USA

E. Waisberg et al. (eds.), *Ophthalmology of Sports*,
https://doi.org/10.1007/978-3-031-88645-4_2

2.1.1 Ocular Injuries in Swimming and Water Polo

Due to their physical nature, water sports such as swimming and water polo can often result in traumatic eye injuries, ranging from accidental finger scratches or pokes to foreign body impact [3]. Water sports-related eye injuries constitute ~3% of all sports-related ocular trauma cases in the US emergency departments from 2010 to 2013 [4]. Recent data from Prevent Blindness in 2020 suggest that eye injuries from water sports are among the most widely reported sports-related eye injuries [5]. Below we discuss the pathophysiology, presentation, and management of ocular trauma as well as miscellaneous vision-related considerations associated with swimming and water polo.

2.1.1.1 Ruptured Globe

Open globes warrant emergent medical and surgical attention, as they are sight-threatening conditions. The sclera covers approximately 80% of the posterior surface of the globe with the cornea covering the remaining 20%. The globe has a few weak points that include the limbus (where the cornea meets the sclera) and the extraocular muscle insertion sites on the sclera (where the sclera is thinnest) [6]. Blunt force trauma (elbow, finger, or ball) onto the globe induces a sudden elevation of intraocular pressure (IOP), making rupture of the globe in the aforementioned locations more likely. A penetrating or perforating injury through the cornea or sclera also leads to compromise of globe integrity [7]. Clinical symptoms of open globe injuries often include severe pain and decreased visual acuity. Clinical signs include presence of prolapsed uveal contents or other intraocular structures (e.g., lens) through a wound, a hyphema, a flat anterior chamber, an irregularly shaped pupil (usually peaking in the direction of the rupture), a low intraocular pressure (IOP), and retinal breaks/tears/detachments, among others [6]. Globe ruptures can sometime be difficult to find, particularly if they are beneath a large dense subconjunctival hemorrhage or if they are posterior. A computed tomography (CT) scan serves as an excellent imaging modality to assess for occult open globe injuries with varied reported sensitivities and specificities [8] as they can also help rule out the presence of an intraocular foreign body, which can affect surgical planning. Ultrasonography can serve in a similar capacity as long as care is taken to avoid application of additional pressure on the unstable globe. Magnetic resonance imaging (MRI) is an option for imaging if a metallic foreign body is not suspected in the injury site. Preoperative management entails placement of an eye shield to protect against further injury, avoiding Valsalva maneuvers (e.g., antiemetics particularly in a nauseous patient), and prophylactic antibiotics (e.g., fluoroquinolone) to prevent endophthalmitis [6]. If there was exposure to a metallic foreign body, ensuring that tetanus vaccination is up to date is critical as well. Definitive management thereafter includes surgical closure of the wound(s) [9].

2.1.1.2 Corneal Injuries

Superficial damage to the cornea can result from fingernail scratches, foreign body impact, or elbow hits, which can be more prominent among those with improper or absent goggle use. A corneal abrasion manifests after the epithelium of the cornea is removed, commonly presenting with eye pain, photophobia, blurred vision, and foreign body sensation in the affected eye. Evaluation entails the application of fluorescein dye to the ocular surface. Shining cobalt blue light allows for identification of the abraded epithelial layer which fluoresces a bright green (Fig. 2.1). Treatment of a corneal abrasion involves the use of topical antibiotic eye drops/ointment, pain control with NSAIDs or acetaminophen [10]. A corneal abrasion can evolve to a corneal infection (keratitis) if not properly monitored and managed. A variety of organisms including (but not limited to) bacteria, fungus, or protozoa can infect the cornea after an abrasion (Fig. 2.2).

2.1.1.3 Conjunctival Injuries

The conjunctiva lines the surface of the sclera and the posterior surfaces of the upper and lower eyelids. A subconjunctival hemorrhage can arise following trauma as noted above, which can result in the accumulation of blood in the subconjunctival space from a ruptured vessel. A recent case report noted barotrauma-related subconjunctival hemorrhage associated with diving [12]. In comparison to the conditions noted above, the patients often have no visual complaints associated with subconjunctival hemorrhage, and symptoms typically spontaneously resolve [13]. Like the cornea, the conjunctiva can become abraded or lacerated. While abrasions and small lacerations are managed with topical antibiotics and close observation, large lacerations should be surgically repaired to avoid the formation of symblepharon. The conjunctiva can also become irritated or injured due to chlorine exposure or rubbing

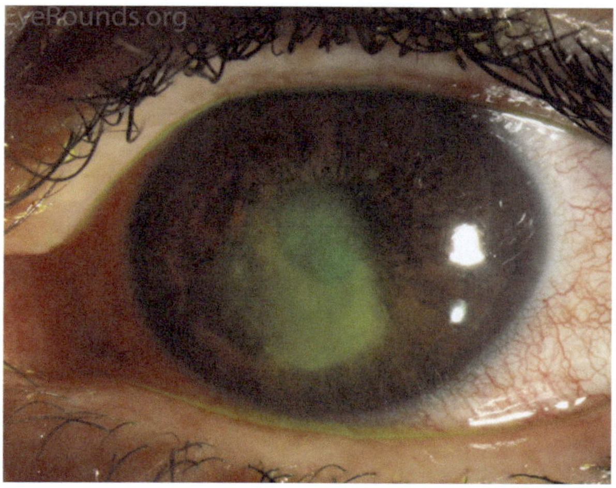

Fig. 2.1 Fluorescein staining showing corneal abrasion. (Image from EyeRounds.org, The University of Iowa and reprinted with permission from Dr. Jesse Vislisel, MD (https://webeye.ophth.uiowa.edu/eyeforum/atlas/pages/corneal-abrasion/corneal-abrasion-LRG.jpg) under Creative Commons License (https://creativecommons.org/licenses/by-nc-nd/3.0/deed.en). (Date accessed Jan 6th, 2025))

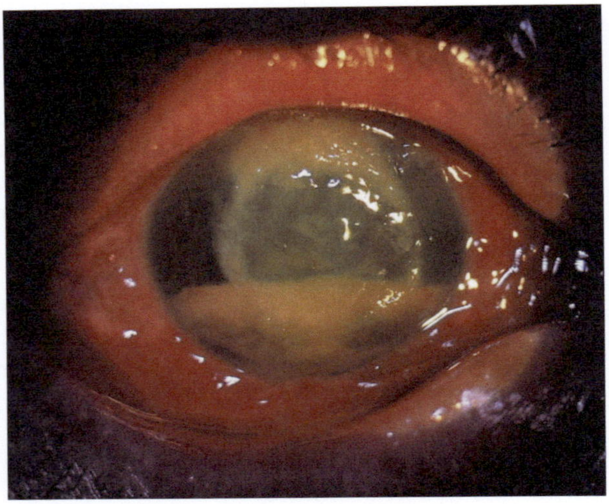

Fig. 2.2 Anterior segment image of a patient with *Acanthamoeba* keratitis. (Image reprinted with permission from Dr. Syed Ahmad under Creative Commons License [11]. (https://creativecommons.org/licenses/by-nc-nd/4.0/). (Date accessed July 10th, 2023))

of the eyes with contaminated hands (chemical conjunctivitis). Infection with a virus or fungus from contaminated pool water has also been reported in association with swimming pool exposure within the past 50 years [14–18]. Lastly, allergic conjunctivitis can also develop following exposure to swimming pool water [11]. Though conjunctivitis is a clinical diagnosis, in some cases laboratory testing and/or cultures can help guide management. The management of conjunctivitis is based on specific etiologies. Bacterial conjunctivitis is often treated empirically with fluoroquinolone drops or polymyxin/trimethoprim drops, while viral conjunctivitis is treated symptomatically with preservative free artificial tears (and rarely with a short course of topical steroid), and lastly allergic and chemical conjunctivitis are treated similarly with topical antihistamine, limiting allergen exposure, and possibly a short course of topical steroid [19].

2.1.1.4 Hyphema

Severe ocular trauma can result in the anterior chamber (AC) bleeding from ruptured vessels in the iris of the ciliary body, as often observed following a shearing force from a water polo or poking finger (Fig. 2.3). Hyphema can range from mild presentation with floating red blood cells to more severe manifestations such as complete filling of the anterior chamber (AC), as reflected in several grading systems [20, 21]. A notable complication of hyphema is elevated intraocular pressure (IOP), most commonly due to clogging of the fine spaces within trabecular meshwork which aids to drain aqueous fluid out of the eye. Over time, untreated elevated intraocular pressure leads to vision loss due to optic nerve atrophy. Furthermore, in cases of hyphema with prolonged elevations of intraocular pressures, corneal blood staining can develop due to red blood cells being pushed into the cornea from the anterior chamber. In some cases, angle recession secondary to injuries to the ciliary

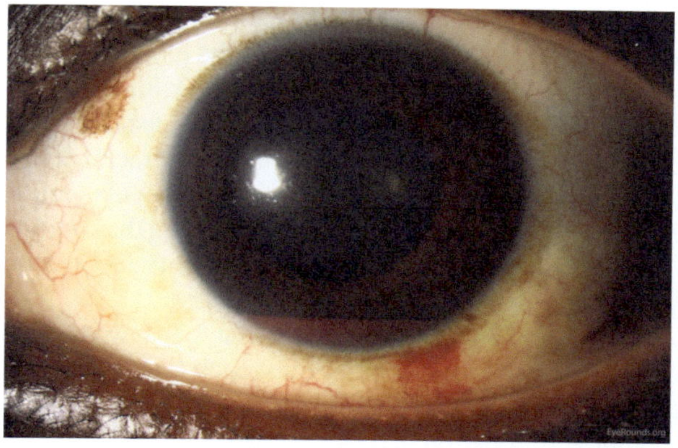

Fig. 2.3 Hyphema of the AC in the eye. (Image from EyeRounds.org, The University of Iowa and reprinted with permission from Dr. Jesse Vislisel, MD (https://webeye.ophth.uiowa.edu/eyeforum/atlas/pages/Hyphema/hyphema-1-LRG.jpg) under Creative Commons License (https://creativecommons.org/licenses/by-nc-nd/3.0/deed.en). (Date accessed Jan 6th, 2025))

body can lead to challenges with the drainage of aqueous from the anterior chamber leading to a form of glaucoma. Importantly, patients with a hyphema warrant close monitoring of intraocular pressure and for the possibility of rebleeding, which can occur as the blood clot retracts and rebleeds within the first 5 days of injury [22, 23].

Due to the sight-threatening nature of hyphema, timely ophthalmic management is necessary. Acute management includes eye shield, head elevation (at least 45 degrees), and bed rest for uncomplicated hyphema [24]. Close monitoring of IOP is warranted, particularly during the first 5 days due to the risk of rebleeding [24]. Pharmacological intervention for hyphema includes topical corticosteroids to reduce inflammation and cycloplegic for those with ciliary spasm, thereby abating the risk of further bleeding. Additionally, topical beta-blockers, prostaglandin analogues, and alpha agonists can be used to manage high IOP. Carbonic anhydrase inhibitors (both topical and oral) can be used, but caution is recommended for treatment in patients with sickle cell disease [22–25]. Hyphema patients could be screened with a sickle prep or hemoglobin electrophoresis. Furthermore, hyphemas that are refractory to medical management may warrant surgical intervention (e.g., anterior chamber wash out filtering surgery (trabeculectomy) or implantation of a glaucoma drainage device) [24].

2.1.1.5 Orbital Fractures

Significant impact to the orbital region during water polo or swimming competition can result in an orbital fracture. Orbital fractures commonly occur in the weakest region of the orbit—the orbital floor (adjacent to the infraorbital canal) or medial wall (thinnest bone of the orbit) [7]. Two main pathophysiologic mechanisms have been used to explain orbital fracture: (1) hydraulic theory, which postulates that elevated intraorbital pressure from retropulsion of the globe results in a fracture via force transmission to the orbital walls, and (2) the buckling theory, which suggests that application of force to the inferior rim directly transmits to the orbital floor, creating a fracture [26]. Clinical presentations of orbital fractures range from bruising and subconjunctival hemorrhage to entrapped extraocular muscle and enophthalmos. The treatment of orbital fractures is contingent on the severity of symptoms: surgery is generally indicated if there is extraocular muscle entrapment or significant enophthalmos [27, 28].

Posterior segment injuries—Severe blunt trauma to the eye, as delineated above, can potentially cause posterior segment injuries, such as retinal tear or detachment. Typical clinical symptoms (e.g., flashes and floaters, visual acuity, or visual field loss) should prompt additional dilated examination of the fundus. Retinal detachment can be managed with surgical intervention such as vitrectomy with gas tamponade and/or scleral buckling, while small retinal tears can be managed with laser photocoagulation. Breaks in Bruch's membrane, the membrane that separates the retina from the choroid, can also be noted in severe traumas. These breaks require monitoring as choroidal neovascular membranes may arise through these breaks over time. In rare cases, central serous chorioretinopathy (CSR) can arise after blunt trauma in the eyes, as recently reported for a case of a water polo player [29].

2.1.1.6 Traumatic Optic Neuropathy

Trauma to the optic nerve from indirect injury secondary to transmitted shock can result in acute injury to the optic nerve. The pathophysiology is thought to be due to shearing of optic nerve's intracanalicular segment, which contributes to further vascular compromise or axonal injury [30]. The severity of traumatic optic neuropathy (TON) can range from mild contusion to complete avulsion, as reported in recent cases of finger-poke injury in a water polo match [31, 32]. On presentation, the optic nerve head may initially appear normal with delayed manifestation of atrophy after several weeks [30]. A relative afferent pupillary defect may be noted on exam. Treatment for TON has remained controversial, ranging from high-dose corticosteroids to surgical optic canal decompression. Literature data have shown a dearth of evidence demonstrating the superiority of any treatment modality in comparison to watchful waiting [33].

Due to these potential injuries, swimming goggles can serve as protective eyewear against not only ocular trauma but also infections and chemical irritations. Swimming goggles, typically composed of polycarbonate, are available in a myriad of lens options ranging from polarized to transitions, thereby enhancing protections against UV light. Given these factors, protective swimming goggles are routinely recommended in swimming and water polo. Despite these benefits, swimming goggles, when associated with improper use or prolonged wear, can lead to various reported ophthalmic conditions with ranging severity, as discussed below.

2.1.1.7 Periorbital Conditions

1. Due to the tight-fitting nature of the goggles exerting pressure in the periorbital region, several types of injuries and irritations have been documented.
   (a) Periorbital dermatitis—Allergic reaction can develop following exposure to the padding from several types of swimming goggles (Fig. 2.4). Many case reports of allergic contact dermatitis secondary to exposure ranging from phenol formaldehyde resin to benzophenone component of swimming goggles have been noted [34–36].
   (b) Periorbital leukoderma—Rare cases of leukoderma have been associated with prolonged swimming goggle use. The hypopigmentation associated with periorbital leukoderma is thought to be due to toxic reaction from neoprene rubber breakdown product [37].
   (c) Periorbital edema and hematoma—Overly tight application of swimming goggles have resulted in a case of eyelid injury, dubbed "purpura gogglorum," characterized by unilateral edematous and purpuric eyelid that resolves with cold compress within 24 h [38].
   (d) Eyelid masses—Several cases of bilateral upper eyelid masses have been noted in competitive swimmers [39–41]. Among these, one report reveals histologic findings suggestive of neuroma [41].
   (e) Supraorbital neuralgia—Prolonged usage of swimming goggles has been associated with supraorbital headache, dubbed swimmer's headache, which is thought to be due to nerve compression in the supraorbital regions. Such diagnosis can be confirmed via nerve block using local anesthesia [42, 43].

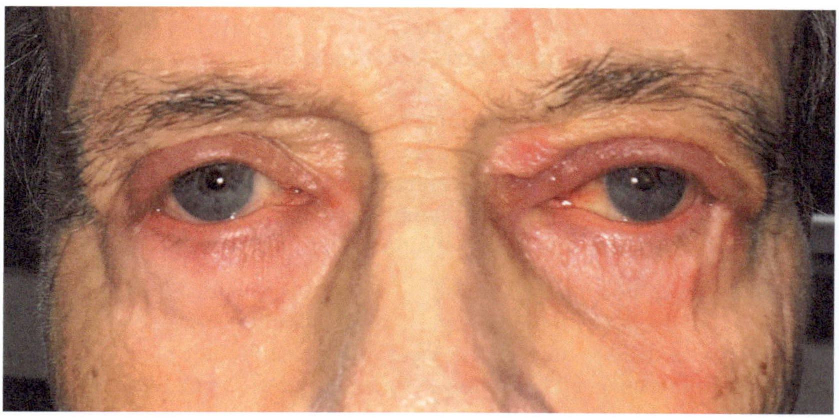

Fig. 2.4 Bilateral periorbital dermatitis. (Image reprinted with permission from Dr. Paul Phelps, MD. (Date accessed Jan 6th, 2025))

2. Anterior segment conditions—Swimming goggles are associated with changes in the anterior segment of varied severity, as discussed below.
   (a) Corneal thinning—Swimming goggle wear is associated with acute and reversible changes in anterior eye segment biometrics such as increased central corneal thinning, which may have implications for patient population with corneal ectasia [44, 45]. Nonetheless, an earlier study examining those with keratoconus showed no evidence demonstrating short-term worsening of corneal parameters [46, 47].
   (b) Corneal erosions—Several case reports of corneal erosion have noted associations with the anti-mist solution of the eyepieces, which was attributed to the alcohol fumes evaporated from the goggles [48, 49].
   (c) Reduction in tear film surface quality break-up time (TFSQ-BUT)—The period between a blink and the initial appearance of dry spots on the cornea is a crucial factor in diagnosing dry eye disease (DED). Reduced TFSQ-BUT has been reported for those wearing swimming goggles, which can be reversed to baseline level following removal [47, 50]. This observation suggests the contribution of swimming goggles to worsening dry eyes, especially for those with existing DED. Nonetheless, swimming goggles do not appear to contribute to known functional changes in the meibomian gland [47].
   (d) Worsening glaucoma drainage bleb—An increase in transconjunctival pressure gradient created by swimming goggles is associated with extension of drainage bleb for a patient who underwent trabeculectomy [51].
   (e) Traumatic corneal injury—Rare cases of traumatic anterior segment injuries (e.g., globe ruptures, hyphema) have been reported for children hitting their eyes with goggles after suddenly pulling the straps [52].
   (f) Increased IOP—Multiple studies have linked increased IOP associated with short-term swimming goggle usage [44, 45, 53–55]. The increased IOP is thought to be attributed to direct mechanical pressure on the orbital tissue, thereby compressing the eyeball. Reassuringly, the increased IOP is reversed following removal of swimming goggles [44, 45, 53]. Further analysis showed that blood flow to the optic nerve head does not appear to significantly change upon wearing swimming goggles [53]. Recent studies demonstrated that regular users of swimming goggles did not have higher incidence of glaucoma compared to non-swimmers [56, 57].

Due to these potential conditions, precautions should be exercised while selecting and using swimming goggles, which should be properly fitted and do not exert excessive pressure on the preorbital areas. Further precaution such as adjusting strap tension and avoiding extended usage of goggles would work well in minimizing the risk of discomfort and potentially serious orbital/periorbital injuries [52].

2.2 Conclusion

In summary, ocular injuries from swimming and water polo can present as a significant source of morbidity for the participants. As such, eye protection such as swimming goggles can significantly reduce the frequency and severity of these discussed ocular injuries. Despite protective measures, rare cases of ocular conditions of varied severity have been associated with swimming goggles, warranting precaution in their selection and proper usage. Continued research and collaboration among health care professionals, sports organizations, and athletes will be essential toward further refining preventive and protective measures against ocular injuries in water sports.

References

1. 2023 USA swimming rules and regulations; 2023. p. 1–133.
2. Understanding the game. USA Water Polo; 2023.
3. Franic M, Ivkovic A, Rudic R. Injuries in water polo. Croat Med J. 2007;48:281–8.
4. Haring RS, Sheffield ID, Canner JK, Schneider EB. Epidemiology of sports-related eye injuries in the United States. JAMA Ophthalmol. 2016;134:1382–90.
5. Sports-related eye injuries by age –2020; 2020.
6. Zhou Y, DiSclafani M, Jeang L, Shah AA. Open globe injuries: review of evaluation, management, and surgical pearls. Clin Ophthalmol. 2022;16:2545–59.
7. Ohana O, Alabiad C. Ocular related sports injuries. J Craniofac Surg. 2021;32:1606–11.
8. Arey ML, Mootha VV, Whittemore AR, Chason DP, Blomquist PH. Computed tomography in the diagnosis of occult open-globe injuries. Ophthalmology. 2007;114:1448–52.
9. Kuhn F, Pelayes DE. Management of the ruptured eye. Eur Ophthalmic Rev. 2009;03:48.
10. Wipperman J, Dorsch J. Evaluation and management of corneal abrasions. Am Fam Physician. 2013;87:114–20.
11. Ahmad SS. Water related ocular diseases. Saudi J Ophthalmol. 2018;32:227–33. https://doi.org/10.1016/j.sjopt.2017.10.009.
12. Ergözen S. Preventable diving-related ocular barotrauma: a case report. Turk J Ophthalmol. 2017;47:296–7.
13. Tarlan B, Kiratli H. Subconjunctival hemorrhage: risk factors and potential indicators. Clin Ophthalmol. 2013;7:1163–70.
14. Bowen AB, Kile JC, Otto C, Kazerouni N, Austin C, Blount BC, Wong HN, Beach MJ, Fry AM. Outbreaks of short-incubation ocular and respiratory illness following exposure to indoor swimming pools. Environ Health Perspect. 2007;115:267–71.
15. Caldwell GG, Lindsey NJ, Wulff H, Donnelly DD, Bohl FN. Epidemic of adenovirus type 7 acute conjunctivitis in swimmers. Am J Epidemiol. 1974;99:230–4.
16. Wang W-Y, et al. Outbreak of microsporidial keratoconjunctivitis associated with water contamination in swimming pools in Taiwan. Am J Ophthalmol. 2018;194:101–9.
17. Schmidt OW, Cooney MK, Foy HM. Adeno-associated virus in adenovirus type 3 conjunctivitis. Infect Immun. 1975;11:1362–70.
18. Heinz F, Bindas B, Cervenka P, Zdebská E. Epidemie plovárenské konjuktivitidy vyvolaná adenovirem typ 3 [epidemics of swimming pool conjunctivitis caused by adenovirus type 3 (author's transl)]. Cesk Epidemiol Mikrobiol Imunol. 1977;25:321–5.
19. Azari AA, Barney NP. Conjunctivitis: a systematic review of diagnosis and treatment. JAMA. 2013;310:1721–30.

20. Read JE, Goldberg MF. Blunt ocular trauma and hyphema. Int Ophthalmol Clin. 1974;14:57–97.
21. Edwards WC, Layden WE, Traumatic hyphema. A report of 184 consecutive cases. Am J Ophthalmol. 1973;75:110–6.
22. Sankar PS, Chen TC, Grosskreutz CL, Pasquale LR. Traumatic Hyphema. Int Ophthalmol Clin. 2002;42:57.
23. Brandt MT, Haug RH. Traumatic hyphema: a comprehensive review. J Oral Maxillofac Surg. 2001;59:1462–70.
24. Walton W, Von Hagen S, Grigorian R, Zarbin M. Management of traumatic hyphema. Surv Ophthalmol. 2002;47:297–334.
25. Woreta FA, et al. Medical interventions for traumatic hyphema. Cochrane Database Syst Rev. 2023;2023:CD005431. https://doi.org/10.1002/14651858.CD005431.pub5.
26. Warwar RE, Bullock JD, Ballal DR, Ballal RD. Mechanisms of orbital floor fractures: a clinical, experimental, and theoretical study. Ophthalmic Plast Reconstr Surg. 2000;16:188.
27. Boyette J, Pemberton J, Bonilla-Velez J. Management of orbital fractures: challenges and solutions. Clin Ophthalmol. 2015;9:2127–37.
28. Gart MS, Gosain AK. Evidence-based medicine: orbital floor fractures. Plast Reconstr Surg. 2014;134:1345.
29. Moschos MM, Gouliopoulos NS. Central serous chorioretinopathy after ocular trauma in the fellow eye during a water-polo game. Case Rep. 2015;2015:bcr2015210779. https://doi.org/10.1136/bcr-2015.
30. Kumaran A, Sundar G, Chye L. Traumatic optic neuropathy: a review. Craniomaxillofac Trauma Reconstr. 2015;8:31–41.
31. Patel TP, Archer EL, Trobe JD. Optic nerve avulsion after finger-poke injury. J Neuroophthalmol. 2018;38:57.
32. Van Brummen A, Mustafi D, Chee YE. Focal retinal ischemia revealed by multimodal imaging after traumatic partial optic nerve avulsion. Retin Cases Brief Rep. 2023;17:70.
33. Wladis EJ, et al. Interventions for indirect traumatic optic neuropathy: a report by the American Academy of Ophthalmology. Ophthalmology. 2021;128:928–37.
34. Melé-Ninot G, et al. Photoallergic contact dermatitis due to benzophenone contained in swimming goggles. Contact Derm. 2020;82:59–60.
35. Azurdia RM, King CM. Allergic contact dermatitis due to phenol-formaldehyde resin and benzoyl peroxide in swimming goggles. Contact Derm. 1998;38:234–5.
36. Vaswani SK, Collins DD, Pass CJ. Severe allergic contact eyelid dermatitis caused by swimming goggles. Ann Allergy Asthma Immunol. 2003;90:672–3.
37. Goette DK. Raccoon-like periorbital leukoderma from contact with swim goggles. Contact Derm. 1984;10:129–31.
38. Jowett NI, Jowett SG. Ocular purpura in a swimmer. Postgrad Med J. 1997;73:819–20.
39. Jordan DR, Gilberg S, Khouri L. Eyelid masses associated with competitive swimming goggles. Can J Ophthalmol. 2001;36:339–40.
40. Ruban J, Mallem M. La paupiere du nageur de competition. J Fr Ophtalmol. 1995;18:426–34.
41. Wirta DL, Dailey RA, Wobig JL. Eyelid neuroma associated with swim goggle use. Arch Ophthalmol. 1998;116:1537–8.
42. O'Brien JC. Swimmer's headache, or supraorbital neuralgia. Baylor Univ Med Cent Proc. 2004;17:418–9.
43. Jacobson R. More goggle headache: supraorbital neuralgia. N Engl J Med. 1983;308:1363.
44. Zhang X, Wang H, Nie Y, Li W. Short-term effects of two types of goggles on intraocular pressure and anterior eye segment biometrics. BMC Ophthalmol. 2022;22:73.
45. Jiménez R, Molina R, García JA, Redondo B, Vera J. Wearing swimming goggles reduces central corneal thickness and anterior chamber angle, and increases intraocular pressure. Curr Eye Res. 2020;45:535–41.
46. Ulusoy DM, Duru Z. Does wearing swimming goggles affect corneal morphology in keratoconic eyes? Arq Bras Oftalmol. 2020;83:225–8.

47. Thomas De Jesus M, et al. A pilot study of the effects of swimming goggles on meibomian glands. Eye Contact Lens. 2022;48:169.
48. Doyle SJ. Acute corneal erosion from the use of anti-misting agent in swimming goggles. Br J Ophthalmol. 1994;78:419.
49. Peng K-L, et al. Corneal injury by anti-misting agent in swim goggles: a case report. Cornea. 2006;25:228.
50. Vera J, Redondo B, Molina R, Jiménez R. Effects of wearing swimming goggles on non-invasive tear break-up time in a laboratory setting. J Optom. 2022;15:154–9.
51. Wakely LA, Reeves G, Ashraff N, Wells AP. Swimming goggles suck. Br J Ophthalmol. 2004;88:1600.
52. Jonasson F. Swimming goggles causing severe eye injuries. Br Med J. 1977;1:881.
53. Ma KT, Chung WS, Seo KY, Seong GJ, Kim CY. The effect of swimming goggles on intraocular pressure and blood flow within the optic nerve head. Yonsei Med J. 2007;48:807–9.
54. Morgan WH, Cunneen TS, Balaratnasingam C, Yu D-Y. Wearing swimming goggles can elevate intraocular pressure. Br J Ophthalmol. 2008;92:1218.
55. Levine B, Radcliffe NM, Starr C. Effects of wearing swimming goggles on intraocular pressure. Invest Ophthalmol Vis Sci. 2007;48:1276.
56. McMonnies CW. The importance of and potential for continuous monitoring of intraocular pressure. Clin Exp Optom. 2017;100:203–7.
57. Franchina M, et al. Swimming goggle wear is not associated with an increased prevalence of glaucoma. Br J Ophthalmol. 2015;99:255.

Chapter 3
Ophthalmic Considerations in Baseball and Softball

Nicholas Panzo, Hamza Memon, Joshua Ong, Daniel M. Laby, and Andrew G. Lee

3.1 Methods

We reviewed the medical literature on ophthalmology in baseball and softball using the following search terms alone and in combination: ophthalmology, sports, baseball, softball, ocular injuries, fastball, sport vision, vision data from the year 1950 to 2023.

Author, Andrew G. Lee, MD, discloses that he has served or is serving as a consultant for the following companies: AstraZeneca, Alexion, Bristol Mayers Squibb, National Football League, Catalyst, Viridian, Ethyreal, NASA, US Department of Justice, Dompe, and Stoke.

N. Panzo (✉) · H. Memon
Texas A&M School of Engineering Medicine, Houston, TX, USA
e-mail: n.panzo@tamu.edu

J. Ong
Department of Ophthalmology and Visual Sciences, University of Michigan Kellogg Eye Center, Ann Arbor, MI, USA

D. M. Laby
SportsVisionNYC/ChampionsEdge, New York, NY, USA

A. G. Lee
Department of Ophthalmology, Blanton Eye Institute, Houston Methodist Hospital, Houston, TX, USA

E. Waisberg et al. (eds.), *Ophthalmology of Sports*,
https://doi.org/10.1007/978-3-031-88645-4_3

3.1.1 Baseball and Softball Basics

3.1.1.1 The Baseball Playing Field

Baseball is played on a diamond-shaped field composed of a 90′ by 90′ infield and an outfield that varies in size. The infield is defined by the first base, second base, third base, and home plate. In Major League Baseball (MLB), the United States and Canadian professional baseball league, each field is unique. The right foul and left foul lines are created by extending a line from home plate along the back of first base and third base, respectively. The outfield is the area inside each foul line and beyond the infield. Figure 3.1 displays the dimensions of a typical baseball field. The MLB has set requirements for the outfield of stadiums built after June 1, 1958, including a minimum distance of 325′ between home plate and the nearest obstruction on the right and left foul line and a 400′ distance between home plate and the nearest obstruction in center field [1]. The pitcher's mound is required to be level with the bases and is 60′ 6″ from home plate. The strike zone is the area over home plate that determines whether a pitch is a strike or a ball. It is a rectangular area above the home plate that comprises the space between the middle of the batter's shoulders and the bottom of their knees [2].

Softball fields vary from baseball fields in their dimension, elevation, and material. Softball fields are smaller than baseball fields with a diamond-shaped field composed of a 60′ by 60′ infield. The outfield requirements are a minimum of 190′ down the foul lines and 235′ in the center. One key difference between baseball and

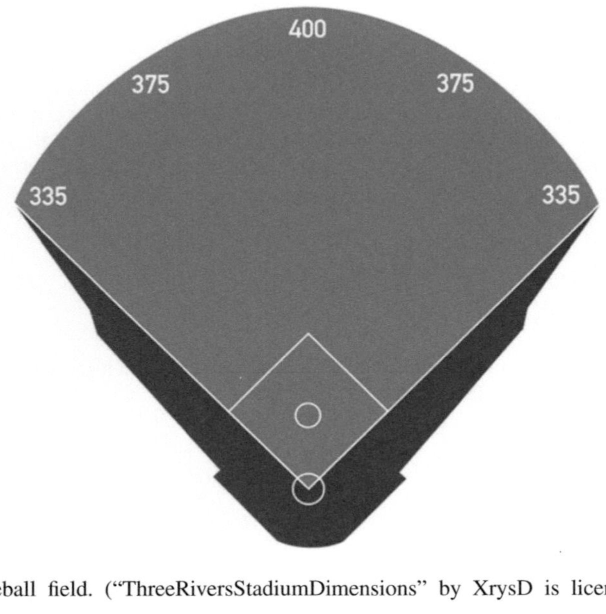

Fig. 3.1 Baseball field. ("ThreeRiversStadiumDimensions" by XrysD is licensed under CC BY-SA 4.0)

softball is the underhanded pitch compared to the overhand baseball pitch. Softball pitchers also throw from a flat surface that is 43′ from home plate.

Since baseball stadiums are not required to have exact dimensions, each ballpark is able to create a unique field that is unlike any other, so long as they follow the aforementioned requirements. These unique features range in purpose from providing tactical advantages to simple aesthetics. The Oakland Coliseum, home of the Oakland A's, has the largest foul territory which is estimated to increase catchable foul pop-ups [3]. Minute Maid Park, home of the Houston Astros, had a small decorative hill at the back of the infield until 2016. These distinctive features differ from the standard fields of many other sports and help create a unique and captivating atmosphere at each stadium.

The visual field of batters also plays a role in the construction of stadiums and is part of the official MLB rules. MLB Rule 1.04 states that it is desirable for the line from home base through the pitcher's plate to second base to run East Northeast [4]. This rule is aimed at reducing the afternoon sun from shining into the batter's eyes, by prioritizing the batter's vision over that of outfielders that may have to catch a pop fly in the afternoon sun. Vision for the batter is further prioritized by the creation of the batter's eye. This is not the eyeball of the batter, but is a term used to refer to the idea that the batter's eye provides a dark and solid contrast from the baseball so the hitter can see the ball approach [5]. Stadiums may also have a large back screen, patch of grass, or other solid background to allow batters to better see the approaching pitch. Figure 3.2 shows one example of the batter's eye and how vision is integral to the design of the field.

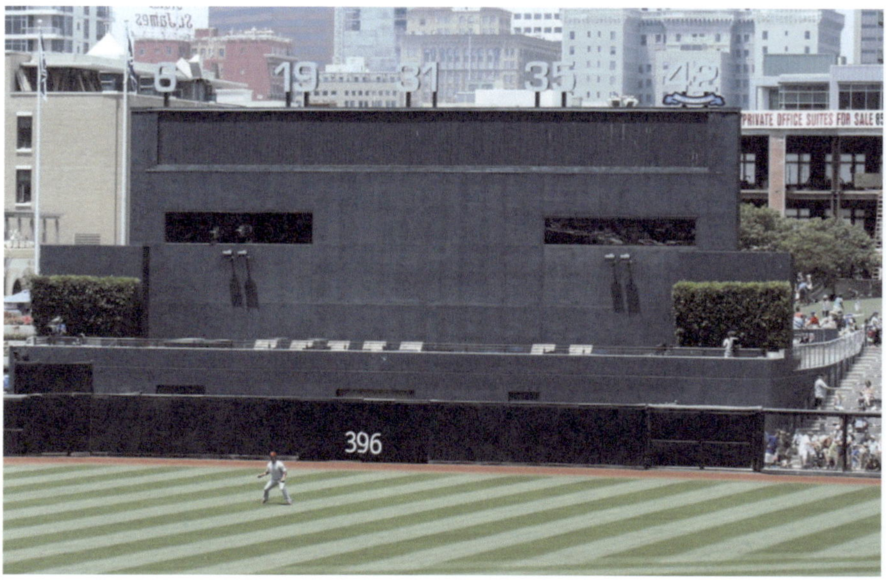

Fig. 3.2 Batter's Eye. ("Batter's Eye" by Jim Epler is licensed under CC BY 2.0)

3.1.1.2 Positions

The defensive positions consist of three outfielders, four infielders, a pitcher, and a catcher. The location of each position is detailed in Fig. 3.3. The infielders are the inner line of defense, responsible for catching any line drives or ground balls and quickly throwing them to the appropriate base before a runner touches that base. The infielders are composed of a first baseman, second baseman, shortstop, and third baseman. The outfielders are the outer line of defense and positioned to catch or field balls that are hit over or through the infield. The outfielders are composed of a left, right, and center fielder. Notably, baseball is one of the few sports in which the defense is responsible for possession of the ball.

On offense, each team's coach sets the batting order before the game which determines the order that players will bat. Each player starts as a hitter and then is designated a base runner if they successfully get on base. The batting order cannot be changed once the game begins, and reserve players must assume the batting order position of the player for whom they substitute. In the following innings, the first batter up is the player who follows the last batter in the previous inning. The batting order is carefully crafted to maximize runs and relies on each player's unique skill set for effective batting.

Different positions in baseball demand a range of specific tasks. For instance, pitchers rely heavily on accuracy and the ability to focus on a precise target, such as the catcher's mitt. On the other hand, outfielders must track the ball as it is hit and maneuver their bodies to make successful catches. Given the distinctive responsibilities associated with each position, researchers have explored potential variations in the visual abilities of pitchers and hitters. In a study conducted by Klemish et al., nine sensorimotor tasks were assessed in both pitchers and hitters, revealing that

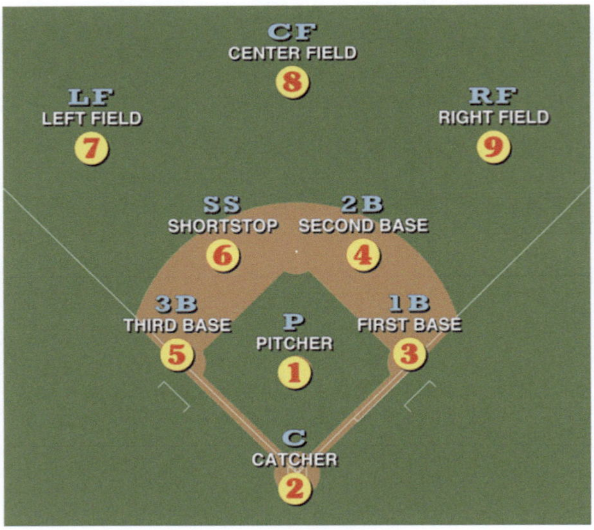

Fig. 3.3 Baseball positions. ("File:Baseball positions.svg" by Michael J is licensed under CC BY-SA 4.0)

professional hitters exhibit better visual acuity and depth perception compared to professional pitchers. This research highlights the unique demands of each baseball position and the essential skills needed to excel at the highest level. While visual perception remains valuable across all positions, its optimization may vary depending on the specific tasks in a given position [6].

3.1.1.3 Game Play

The primary goal of baseball is to score more runs than the other team in the given set of innings. Baseball consists of nine innings, and softball consists of seven innings. Each inning is further divided into the top, or first half, and bottom, or second half, of each inning. At the start of the game, the away team will take the offensive position and bat first, and then the teams switch once the offensive team has recorded three outs. An out occurs when either a defensive player tags a baserunner with the ball, the baserunner fails to reach the base before the defensive player with the ball does, a ball hit by the batter is caught, or the batter swings at three pitches without making contact with the ball. A foul ball is a ball that is hit by the batter and goes outside the foul lines [7]. A foul ball on the first or second pitch is counted as an out. However, on the third pitch, a foul is still counted as a foul but results in another pitch. Players cannot get out on a foul unless a defensive player catches the ball [8].

Scoring is based on runs, which occur when a batter progresses around the bases, ultimately returning to home plate. A team can receive up to four points on an at-bat if the bases are loaded, meaning a baserunner at first, second, and third base. If the game is tied after all the innings are played, extra innings are played until one team has the lead at the end of a full inning.

Baseball and softball rely heavily on visual perception throughout the game. Whether on offense or defense, players constantly observe and react to the ball. The complex assessments, movements, and decisions executed by each player require precise information gathered through their vision. In essence, the accuracy and efficiency of players' visual processing play a pivotal role in the swift and strategic maneuvers of these sports.

3.1.1.4 Equipment

The two most basic and essential pieces of baseball equipment are the baseball bat and baseball. A regulation baseball is approximately three inches in diameter and weighs roughly 5 ounces. The baseball core consists of a cork center with two yarn wrappings and a layer of horsehide [9]. Baseball bats are composed of wood or hollow metals such as aluminum, although the MLB requires that the bat be composed of one piece of solid wood. Similar to baseball, softball requires a softball and softball bat. Softballs are approximately 4 inches in diameter with a cork center, leather or rubber coat, and yarn seams [10]. Softball bats are composed of a hollow metal such as aluminum and have a thicker barrel than baseball bats, which help make contact with the larger ball size.

Baseball players will also frequently use "eye black," a greasy material or strip worn under both eyes. The eye black is used to reduce glare on a sunny day, which can be particularly helpful for outfielders catching a fly ball. Although there remains some skepticism regarding the effectiveness of eye black, research has demonstrated its effectiveness. One study used a contrast chart on 46 participants to evaluate the effectiveness of eye black and found that eye black grease reduces glare and improves contrast sensitivity [11]. Whether it is believed to be a psychological intimidation factor, or a true aid in vision, eye black is commonly used in many outdoor American sports and remains a staple of baseball culture.

3.1.1.5 Statistics

It would be remiss to describe baseball without discussing baseball statistics. They are used to evaluate players, develop gameplay strategy, and sometimes rank players. This general terminology is used by fans and analysts and is helpful when discussing the performance of players. For hitters, batting average and runs batted in (RBI) are two major statistics. Batting average is determined by dividing a player's hits from at-bats [12]. RBI is the amount of times a batter's appearance at bat has resulted in a run being scored. For pitchers, earned run average (ERA) and walks plus hits per inning pitched (WHIP) are commonly used to evaluate pitchers. ERA is the earned runs a pitcher allows per nine innings [13].

One emerging statistic is the use of vision data and visual scoring. Kirschen and Laby evaluated vision data from six major league teams, collecting data on 759 players. The data was analyzed retrospectively using a grading rubric to grade the visual readiness of prospects for the MLB. The results showed that players with higher vision grades were more likely to be drafted than players with lower grades. This research suggests vision data can be used to aid in the selection of players and gauge their ability to perform at higher levels [14]. As the field grows, there is potential to use this metric at other levels of play and aid in player selection and performance.

3.1.2 Ocular Trauma Epidemiology

As players step up to the plate, their feet can be as close as six inches to home plate with their arms, knees, and head even closer to the future target of a 90 mph fastball. Batters are at risk of being hit each pitch, and in the MLB, the number of hit by pitches has been increasing [15]. At any level, there is inherent risk of stepping into the batter's box and facing down a fastball, but other positions are also at risk of ocular trauma. After a hitter makes contact with the ball, it travels towards the pitcher into the outfield. The fast speed of a baseball and explosive hitting power of batters mean that everyone from players, coaches, and even fans need to be attentive of the ball's location.

In a study that investigated ocular injuries in the MLB over the course of a year, there were 21 recorded eye injuries with the majority, 52%, occurring from contact with a batted ball [16]. Of the batted ball injuries, 54% occurred to players at bat, 27% to players/coaches on the sideline, and 18% to players in the infield. The most common symptom players experienced was decreased vision in players' left eye. Eye injuries due to sliding, collision with other players, or dirt in their eyes were also reported as injuries. The occurrence of ocular injuries in baseball is more prevalent among pediatric and recreational players than at the professional level. This can be attributed to the larger population of youth players in contrast to the smaller number of professional players. Despite the higher pitching and batting speeds in professional baseball, the overall incidence of ocular injuries appears to be lower in this group.

In 2019, baseball and softball had the most participation of any team sport in the USA, with 25.6 million participants [17]. While these numbers have declined, baseball and softball remain one of the most popular team sports in the USA. In 2021, baseball was the second most played team sport for children aged 6–17 years old in the United States and softball was the fifth most played sports for high school girls [18]. Due to the large number of players in the USA, and inherent risks associated with the sport, baseball is the second leading cause of ocular injury in male patients [19]. In female patients, baseball or softball is reported to be the most common cause of ocular injury [14]. There are estimated 86,146 baseball and 51,112 softball injuries annualy among children aged 7–21 years old [20]. On average, there are 2,900 emergency department visits due to baseball or softball related eye injuries [21].

A 2022 NEISS study found that ocular injuries related to baseball are mostly due to contact with the ball in a recreational setting and result in blurry vision. Contusions and abrasions are the most common diagnoses accounting for 45.8% of ocular injuries followed by other injuries (e.g., foreign body and unspecified injury (36%), hyphema (8.5%), Iritis/iridocyclitis (6%), lid laceration (1.7), ruptured globe (0.8%), retinal injury (0.4%), and orbital fracture (0.2%). Visual sequelae resulted in blurry vision, vision loss, other sequelae including anisocoria, diplopia, and non-specific visual disturbances, followed by photosensitivity [22].

The American Academy of Ophthalmology and the American Academy of Pediatrics have classified baseball and softball as high-risk activities along with paintball, basketball, and ice hockey, in total accounting for 55% of eye-injuries in the USA. Ocular injuries can have severe consequences, including blindness and vision loss, often necessitating the involvement of an ophthalmologist to assess their severity. Sports-related ocular injuries alone account for approximately 13,500 cases of legal blindness yearly [23]. Therefore, it is crucial to be aware of the risks associated with sports activities and prioritize the use of appropriate protective gear to prevent such injuries. It is important to note that overall baseball is considered a safe sport with major injuries occurring 72% less frequently than in football, 23% less likely in boys soccer, and 20% less likely than in boys basketball.

3.1.2.1 Contusion/Abrasions

Almost half of the ocular injuries in baseball are contusions/abrasions. An abrasion is the result of corneal epithelium damage, typically caused by rubbing the eye or coming into contact with equipment like a ball, bat, or glove. Because this sensitive layer of the eye is also prone to damage from relatively non-traumatic causes, abrasions should be considered even if a patient does not recall any traumatic event [24]. Patients with corneal abrasions may present with pain, tearing, blurred vision, photophobia, and foreign body sensation [25]. Abrasions are most frequently invisible without magnification and therefore require fluorescein staining with slit lamp examination for proper diagnosis. Treatment for corneal abrasions should aim to protect against infections and relieve pain. Antibiotic drops can be used to reduce risk of infection, and NSAIDs or Tylenol can be used for pain relief. Most corneal abrasions are self-limited, but conservative symptomatic treatment and referral to an eye care provider are recommended.

Contusions are the result of blunt force to either the periocular tissues, or the eye directly and typically present with a bruise around the eye, pain, or visual disturbances [26]. All contusions may be associated with orbital bone fractures and more serious ocular contusions. Orbital contusions occur due to blunt forces impacting the globe directly, or indirectly by forces that penetrate the bony rim of the orbit. Contusions can cause iritis, hyphema, increased intraocular pressure, retinal damage and should be referred to an ophthalmologist for diagnosis and medical or surgical therapy. If examination of an orbital/periorbital contusion does not reveal further injury, then a cold compress can be used to reduce swelling.

3.1.2.2 Foreign Body

Foreign body injuries are the result of any foreign body within the orbit, either penetrating or non-penetrating. We will focus on non-penetrating foreign body diagnosis as this is most common in baseball. Dirt, dust, or clay can get into the eye of players as they slide for a base, but these small particles typically do not necessitate an emergency. Other foreign bodies, including glass or metal, can become embedded in the eye and lead to further damage and irritation [21]. Players should refrain from rubbing their eyes and instead blink and then rinse their eyes with saline or tap water. An ophthalmologist should be consulted if the object is not removed from the eye after the eyewash or if there is continued irritation.

3.1.2.3 Hyphema

Hyphema is the accumulation of red blood cells in the anterior chamber of the eye which can fill the entire anterior chamber obscuring the iris and pupil (8-ball hyphema). However, many hyphemas may be microscopic and barely visible without slit lamp examination. Traumatic forces can compress the globe and injure the iris, ciliary body, trabecular meshwork, creating shearing forces that tear blood vessels in these tissues and lead to accumulation of blood in the anterior chamber [27]. Any degree of hyphema is evidence of ocular contusion and should initiate further evaluation by an ophthalmologist for more serious ocular damage. Over 50% of all sport-related cases of hyphema are a result of racquet sports, baseball, and softball [28]. Common symptoms from traumatic hyphema are blurry vision, headache, eye pain, or photophobia.

The primary initial goal for hyphema treatment is to shield the eye from further trauma. Initial evaluation and treatment by ophthalmology is recommended (e.g., shielding the eye, reducing activity levels, and elevating the head). Due to the potential risk for bleeding, pain management should include acetaminophen (Tylenol) and not aspirin or nonsteroidal anti-inflammatory drugs (NSAIDs). Patients should be monitored by an ophthalmologist. Rebleeding occurs in up to 38% of traumatic hyphema cases 3–5 days following injury [29]. Surgery is rarely need, but markedly elevated intraocular pressure or corneal blood straining may require more aggressive treatment. Return to play will be determined by an ophthalmologist and patients can expect to wait 1–2 weeks before competing again [23].

3.1.2.4 Iritis/Iridocyclitis

Traumatic uveitis is characterized by inflammation that affects the iris, ciliary body, or choroid in the eye. Among its various forms, anterior uveitis, also known as iritis, primarily involves inflammation of the iris located at the front of the eye and is the most prevalent type. Another subtype, iridocyclitis, involves inflammation of both the iris and ciliary body. Blunt trauma to the eye can result in traumatic iritis, which accounts for 20% of iritis cases and is suspected to be the major form of baseball-related iritis. Blunt trauma to the eye can cause cellular damage and initiate an inflammatory response within the anterior chamber. This inflammatory response triggers the release of prostaglandins, which can lead to necrosis of the iris/ciliary body, resulting in increased vascular permeability, accompanied by elevated levels of white blood cells and protein.

Patients with uveitis may present with unilateral photophobia, decreased vision, redness, or pain [30]. Slit lamp examination will reveal white blood cells/protein in the anterior chamber, known as “cell and flare” [31]. Traumatic iritis is generally self-limiting and resolves within 7–14 days. Topical cycloplegics can be used to reduce ciliary and pupillary spasm, reducing patient pain and discomfort [32]. Additionally, topical corticosteroids can be administered to reduce potential complications associated with inflammation [20]. Follow-up examinations are recommended 1 week after the trauma to assess the reduction of inflammation and to gradually taper off the steroids. Another follow-up appointment should be scheduled after a month to ensure there is no relapse of the condition.

3.1.2.5 Laceration

Lacerations are a cut to the eye and can involve the eyelid, conjunctiva, or cornea. The deeper the penetration, the more potential there is for vision loss; therefore, determination of the depth of the laceration is essential. Corneal lacerations result from injury to the cornea and affect deeper layers than abrasions. If a laceration penetrates through the entire layer of the cornea, it may rupture the globe. Lacerations commonly occur when a sharp object hits the eye but can also result from blunt trauma, which would typically occur in a baseball setting. The extent of vision damage depends on the depth of the injury and any potential inflammation that results from this injury. Lacerations that involve the Bowman's layer or deeper may result in corneal scarring and a reduction in visual clarity [33].

Patients with corneal or conjunctival lacerations may present with decreased vision, severe pain, tearing, or bleeding in the eye. A seidel test, which utilizes fluorescent dye and a slit lamp, can be used to identify if the laceration is full-thickness and determine if there is an ocular leak [34]. An assessment of the globe should be completed when patients present with eyelid lacerations. If there is no damage to the globe, then proper wound debridement and surgical repair can begin [35]. Players with a suspected corneal laceration should refrain from rinsing with water, removing any penetrating object, rubbing their eye, applying pressure to the eye, or taking NSAIDs, which may increase bleeding [36]. Corneal laceration is a serious injury that usually requires surgery to close the eye and prevent infection [31]. For penetrating injuries, it may be necessary to remove the foreign object that remains in the eye.

3.1.2.6 Ruptured Globe

Although ruptured globes account for less than 1% of ocular-related baseball injuries, it represents a severe injury, and therefore, this section will discuss some key features of the injury. Severe blunt trauma has the potential to significantly elevate intraocular pressure, reaching a level that can cause the eyewall to rupture, leading to a condition known as a ruptured globe. The inside-out force created from a ruptured globe will frequently result in tissue herniations and occurs at the weakest point on the globe [37]. The location of the rupture commonly occurs behind the insertion of the rectus muscles in patients without a history of intraocular surgery and at the previous incision site for patients with prior surgery [38].

Surgery is necessary to repair the damage to the globe, and delays in surgical care can increase the risk of choroidal hemorrhage, which is the most serious complication of open-globe injury [39]. Antiemetics can be administered to reduce the risk of increased intraocular pressure as well as prophylactic antibiotic treatment [40]. Postoperative follow-up is typically scheduled at 1 day, 1 week, 1 month, and 3 months after surgery [35]. Prior visual acuity, wound location, wound length, mechanism of injury, retinal, detachment, and vitreous hemorrhage all play a role in predicting the final visual acuity after ruptured globe injury [41].

3.1.3 Eye Protection

It is estimated that 90% of sports-related eye injuries can be prevented with adequate eye protection, yet ocular injuries are one of the major sources of debilitation in the United States and can have lasting physical, emotional, and economic impacts [17, 42]. Protective measures have been implemented throughout professional baseball history. Unfortunately, many of these safety implementations come at the cost of payers suffering serious injuries that push the league to make safety changes. In 1967, outfielder Tony Conigliaro was hit by a fastball, suffering a fracture to his orbital and zygomatic bone, leading him to ultimately retire due to significant visual impairment [43]. It was not until 1971 when batting helmets became mandatory, and 1983 for the MLB to require one ear flap. After the death of a Rockies minor league first base coach in 2007, the MLB required base coaches to wear batting helmets [44].

While traditional baseball helmets provide protection to the cranial bones, there is minimal protection to the facial bones, including bones that create the orbit. One of the more recent advances, which may decrease facial/ocular injuries, is the C-Flap extension. The C-Flap, originally designed in the 1980s, is a protective plastic that attaches to batting helmets and extends over the cheek and jaw [45]. This extension is mainly used to protect the jaw of batters but may also provide additional protection to the orbit. Further studies are required to validate the ocular protective properties of these guards. The use of this equipment has increased in recent years at the professional level but has not gained sufficient traction in youth leagues because these extensions do not meet National Operating Committee on Standards for Athletic Equipment (NOCSAE) standards. The National Federation of State High School Associations (NFHS) requires that batters, baserunners, on-deck batters wear a batting helmet that meets NOCSAE standards, which the C-Flap extension does not. Currently, there is a lack of data for the safety and efficacy of C-flaps for preventing ocular injury and should not be considered eye protection for baseball.

Advances in ocular safety measures for youth baseball are continuously being discussed. The two major pieces of equipment that have been developed and implemented are helmets with protective face shields and low-impact baseballs [46]. Currently, these are not required for little league players but are listed as optional equipment [47]. The only ocular protective equipment that is required is for the catcher, who must wear a catcher's helmet that covers the face and provides ocular protection from balls or bats. Players who wear glasses are recommended to wear safety glasses. Base runners and batters are required to wear helmets that cover both ears. There are no facemask requirements for high-school or National Collegiate Athletic Association (NCAA) baseball.

The NFHS mandated in 2005 that fast-pitch softball batting helmets must have NOCSAE-approved faceguards [48]. This change has increased the acceptance of faceguards in softball, and although there are currently no national rules on protective face guards for outfielders, several states have implemented a facemask requirement for in-field positions [49–51]. Faceguards have been shown to be effective in reducing the incidence of oculofacial injuries [52]. However, it is worth noting that in collegiate-level NCAA softball, players are not mandated to wear face masks.

Baseball and softball players are at risk of ocular injuries from batted balls, pitches, and throws. Proper eye protection can greatly reduce the risk of ocular injury. Although baseball has created guards to protect the face of players, they are not sufficient to protect the orbit and eye. Players who wear prescription glasses should request prescription protective sports eyewear to fully protect their eye. Sports safety glasses should meet the American society for testing and materials (ASTM) and American national standards institute (ANSI) safety standards to be fully qualified for sports activities. Face guards that meet NOCSAE standards are also sufficient to protect the eye from contact with the ball. If the proper eye protection is implemented players can reduce ocular injury without reducing visual clarity.

3.1.4 Performance and Vision

With pitching speeds reaching up to 108 mph, batters often have less than 400 ms before the ball is in the catcher's glove. This is without taking into account the 150 ms visuo-motor required to swing the bat toward the ball, giving the batter 250 ms to track the ball, identify the pitch, decide to swing, and begin the muscle contraction needed to make contact [53]. With such a short time to react, it is no wonder that the average batting average is 0.250, meaning less than 3 out of 10 pitches will be hit.

The complex visual pathway necessary to pitch, hit, throw, or catch a baseball relies on dynamic visual acuity (DVA), static visual acuity (SVA), smooth pursuit, and saccades. These features of eye movement enable players to effectively track the ball from the pitcher's hand and accurately anticipate its trajectory, allowing them to make informed decisions on whether to swing and make contact if the ball is predicted to fall within the strike zone. SVA is the ability to distinguish details of objects that are stationary. DVA is the ability to visualize objects when there is relative movement between the subject and the object [54]. Having an enhanced DVA allows batters and fielders to properly visualize pitches and hits and may increase the chance of getting a hit on base or completing a catch in baseball. Researchers have found a link between DVA and expertise across many sports, highlighting the connection between visual and athletic performance [49]. Both SVA and DVA have been found to be greatly increased in professional baseball players compared to the general public [55, 56].

Saccades allow the eyes to quickly move between two points of focus at speeds of over a hundred degrees per second [57, 58]. This rapid alternation in fixation allows for quick shifts of attention from one point to another, but it can also temporarily suppress vision due to the rapid movement of the eye. This is termed "saccadic suppression" and can extend 20 ms after the saccadic movement [59]. On the other hand, smooth pursuits, which are slower eye movements, enable the smooth tracking of objects at a speed of up to 100° per second [60, 61]. Smooth pursuit is utilized as outfielders track a ball going into the outfield, a ground ball across the infield, or even the first portion of the pitch as it travels toward the batter. This slow pursuit allows for clarity and foveation across the ball's path. The vestibulo-ocular reflex keeps the eyes focused on an object as players' heads move. This allows for players to rotate their head as they track a pitch while keeping focus on the ball.

Many studies have investigated ball tracking during a baseball pitch, investigating the complex eye, body, and head movements required to properly assess and hit a pitch. Predicting the pitch is the first step in properly hitting the ball and relies on an understanding of strategy as well as visual cues. Experienced players will focus on the pitcher's arm or ball release point, while less experienced players focus closer to the midline of the pitcher's body upon pitch release [62]. Experienced players also move their eyes slower and with a reduced distribution of area than novice players during the pitcher's throw, indicating that advanced players use peripheral vision to evaluate the pitcher and the ball trajectory [63].

After a pitch is released, players are able to gauge the time to contact using the ratio of current retinal image size of the ball to the rate of change in the ball's retinal image size [64]. Visualizing the rotation of the seams is useful for predicting the rotation, which provides an additional cue to estimate time to contact and determine the type of pitch [65].

As the ball approaches the batter, head and eye movements are used to track the ball. Kishita et al. analyzed the combination of eye and head movement to investigate how players track the pitch at different ball speeds. Eye and head movement are involved in tracking pitches and happen at two different portions of time. In the first half of the pitch, head movement will be larger, while eye movements will employ smooth pursuit. In the second half of the pitch as the range of motion for the eyes and head increase, eye movement can increase to up to 100° per second, initiating the saccadic predictive motion of the eyes. When the ball is five feet from the plate, it travels 3 times faster than the fastest human can track and provides little value to the batter [66]. As pitch speed increases, the initiation of the saccadic movement begins earlier in the ball path. It has been found that the timing of the anticipatory saccades are influenced by the expertise of players and the predictability of pitches [67]. Given the short duration of the pitch and normal muscle contraction latencies, it is unlikely that any visual information perceived during the latter portions of the pitch can be utilized to change muscle contraction or bat position and trajectory.

At the professional level, the speed of the pitched ball exceeds saccadic movement. As a result, and as noted above, it has been found that the visual system focuses on a point dozens of feet from the plate during contact [68]. The final fixation point before athletes initiate movement, termed the "quiet eye" by Dr. Joan Vickers of the University of Calgary, is a key component in many sports. It has been well-researched across a variety of sports, including basketball and golf, where players have been analyzed based on their focal points before contact and their success in putting or making a free throw. These studies have found that maintaining fixation before and after initiating movement improves performance [69, 70]. While the theory of quiet eye and performance has been focused on aiming sports such as golf, basketball, and archery, there has been research into the quiet eye in softball performance. One study investigated the effects of over-speed video training on pitch recognition in collegiate softball players and found that both over-speed and regular video training can improve quiet eye duration and pitch recognition [71]. Similar to the focus of elite players on the release point of the ball during the pitch, it appears that the quiet eye can improve the ability of players to detect a pitch and initiate appropriate movement. Although the old adage of "keeping your eye on the ball" may not be possible as ball speeds increase, the ability to visualize and predict ball movement in order to accurately hit a pitch relies on many ophthalmologic as well as visuo-cognitive principles.

3.1.5 Visual Training

Vision is a critical factor in sports performance, and many visual metrics have been shown to correlate with improved athlete performance. For example, a study by Laby et al. found a statistically significant relationship between visual function and batting performance in 585 professional baseball players [72]. Additionally, improved eye-hand visual-motor reaction time, which is the connection between visual input and motor movements, has also been shown to significantly correlate with improved batting performance [73, 74].

Early research into the success of batters and eye movements suggested that improved performance can be linked to faster smooth-pursuit, suppression of the vestibulo-ocular reflex, and use of anticipatory saccade [54]. Further studies have linked visual reaction time to increased batting averages [75]. Studies on ocular dominance and hand dominance have linked successful batting with central ocular dominance and crossed eye-hand dominance, but it remains unclear if these studies are valid due to lack of consistent clinical tests for measuring ocular dominance and the complex binocular processing that occurs when both eyes are open [76, 77].

Due to the connection between vision and baseball performance, many studies have aimed to create protocols and training programs to improve players' visual and on-field performance. As is true for any nascent specialty, there is a wide range of scientific reports available in the medical literature. In a 2021 publication, Laby and Appelbaum presented a critical review of published studies that attempt to link visual assessment and training to sports performance. They noted that although there appeared to be promising evidence to support the approach that visual assessment and training in this area can lead to improved competitive sports performance, additional methodological improvement in study design, execution, analysis, and reporting is needed in this growing field [78].

In all sports, the goal of visual training is to allow players to make the appropriate decision based on the least amount of information, with the least amount of effort [79]. Different programs have been proposed to improve the visual function of baseball players including computer programs, watching faster pitches, or

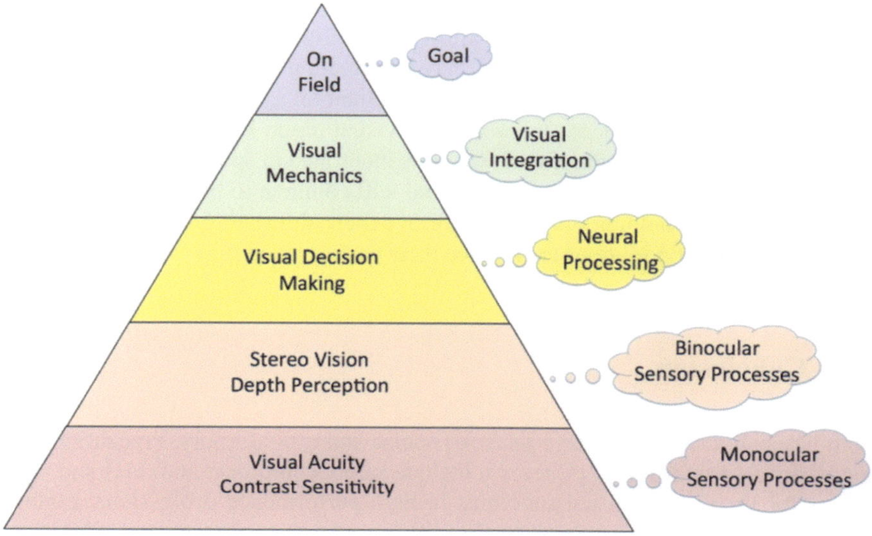

Fig. 3.4 Sports vision pyramid. (Copyright 2009, EYEcheck Systems, LLC used with permission)

tracking the color of stickers on pitched balls [80, 81]. One study created an optic training plan consisting of targeting gabor patches and resulted in improved vision, lower strikeouts, more runs created [82]. The use of dynamic visual training has shown to improve players' hit distance and launch angle [83]. Although these programs improve individual metrics, other programs have aimed at creating a more extensive program to improve performance.

In order to develop a comprehensive sports vision training program, Laby and Kirschen have developed the sports vision pyramid (Fig. 3.4), which outlines the visual elements that must be built upon for optimal performance [84]. At the bottom of the pyramid is visual acuity and contrast sensitivity representing visual abilities unique to each eye alone. Above this level is binocular visual function and stereoscopic vision that creates depth and three-dimensional shapes. After these first two levels, a decision is made from the visual input. At the plate, this represents the decision to swing or not swing at a pitch and is intrinsically reliant on the visual information and predictions that the batter has created. Once a decision is made then the next level, visual mechanics, uses the visual information to initiate a visually guided and timed motor movement.

The pyramid allows players to evaluate their visual performance, systematically, at increasing levels to achieve maximal performance. Each of the lower levels of the pyramid must be satisfied first, in order to move up to the next level. For example, a player with 20/40 vision could most improve their performance by correcting the lowest level of the pyramid, visual acuity, and contrast sensitivity, before improving their visual decision-making. It is worth noting that the visual processing system that occurs in our brains is more complicated than the visual pyramid, but the pyramid represents a simplified two-dimensional approach to understanding sports vision. Other models, such as the artificial intelligence multi-nodal approach, described many weighted nodes that relay information to each other [79]. In this network, the decision to initiate movement is reliant on a variety of different inputs such as previous experiences, emotions, and visual input. Both paradigms provide valuable insight into how the visual system is integrated in sports performance. The field of sports vision training is growing and will continue to be a valuable tool for players and teams, helping players to improve their ability to process and respond to visual information in order to enhance their performance [85].

3.2 Conclusion

Both baseball and softball have risks for ocular and orbital injury. Precautions and countermeasures for injury protection include safety equipment and rules and regulations for the games. Visual functions in high performance professional athletes include enhanced predictive saccade and pursuit eye movements, SVA, and DVA. Visual training to enhance player performance has been proposed in these sports, but further work is necessary to determine their efficacy and validity.

References

1. Field Dimensions. MLB.com. https://www.mlb.com/glossary/rules/field-dimensions. Accessed 14 Oct 2023.
2. Strike Zone. MLB.com. https://www.mlb.com/glossary/rules/strike-zone. Accessed 14 Oct 2023.
3. Fink D. MLB: Marco Estrada is the king of the foul pop-up. Beyond the Box Score. https://www.beyondtheboxscore.com/2019/2/17/18226338/mlb-marco-estrada-oakland-athletics-foul-pop-ups. Published 17 Feb 2019. Accessed 14 Oct 2023.
4. 2010 Official baseball rules. MLB.com. https://mlb.mlb.com/mlb/downloads/y2010/official_rules/2010_OfficialBaseballRules.pdf. Accessed 11 Nov 2023.
5. Travis Coverstonatter's. Batter's eye: baseball terminology. https://www.thebaseballjournal.com/terminology/batters-eye-baseball-terminology/ March 25, 2015. Accessed 11 Nov 2023.
6. Klemish D, Ramger B, Vittetoe K, Reiter JP, Tokdar ST, Appelbaum LG. Visual abilities distinguish pitchers from hitters in professional baseball. J Sports Sci. 2018;36(2):171–9. https://doi.org/10.1080/02640414.2017.1288296.
7. Foul Ball. MLB.com. https://www.mlb.com/glossary/rules/foul-ball. Accessed 14 Oct 2023.
8. Foul Tip. MLB.com. https://www.mlb.com/glossary/rules/foul-tip. Published (if available). Accessed 14 Oct 2023.
9. Coatess A. Author(s). How big is a baseball? Wezen-Ball. https://wezen-ball.com/how-big-is-a-baseball/#The_History_of_Baseball. Published 2 Oct 2023. Accessed 14 Oct 2023.
10. What is softball made of? Rookie Road. https://www.rookieroad.com/softball/what-is-softball-made/. Accessed 14 Oct 2023.
11. DeBroff BM, Pahk PJ. The ability of periorbitally applied antiglare products to improve contrast sensitivity in conditions of sunlight exposure. Arch Ophthalmol. 2003;121(7):997–1001. https://doi.org/10.1001/archopht.121.7.997.

12. Batting Average. MLB.com. https://www.mlb.com/glossary/standard-stats/batting-average. Accessed 14 Oct 2023.
13. Earned Run Average. MLB.com. https://www.mlb.com/glossary/standard-stats/earned-run-average. Accessed 14 Oct 2023.
14. Kirschen DG, Laby DM. The uses of vision data in selecting players for the major league baseball draft. Optom Vis Sci. 2021;98(7):809–14. https://doi.org/10.1097/OPX.0000000000001736.
15. Treder S. The hbp explosion that almost nobody seems to have noticed. FanGraphs. https://tht.fangraphs.com/the-hbp-explosion-that-almost-nobody-seems-to-have-noticed/. January 30, 2007. Accessed 14 Oct 2023.
16. Zagelbaum BM, Hersh PS, Donnenfeld ED, Perry HD, Hochman MA. Ocular trauma in major-league baseball players. N Engl J Med. 1994;330(14):1021–3. https://doi.org/10.1056/NEJM199404073301421.
17. Kelly M. Baseball participation increases. MLB.com. https://www.mlb.com/news/baseball-participation-increases. Published 20 Feb 2019. Accessed 14 Oct 2023.
18. Aspen Institute. State of play: 2022 national youth sports participation trends; 2022. Retrieved from: www.aspeninstitute.org/wp-content/uploads/2022/11/2022_SoP_National_ParticipationTrends.pdf.
19. Haring RS, Sheffield ID, Canner JK, Schneider EB. Epidemiology of sports-related eye injuries in the United States. JAMA Ophthalmol. 2016;134(12):1382–90. https://doi.org/10.1001/jamaophthalmol.2016.4253.
20. Farooqi AS, Lee A, Abreu E, Talwar D, Maguire KJ. Epidemiology of pediatric baseball and softball player injuries. Orthop J Sports Med. 2021;9(12):23259671211052585. Published 15 Dec 2021. https://doi.org/10.1177/23259671211052585.
21. Miller KN, Collins CL, Chounthirath T, Smith GA. Pediatric sports- and recreation-related eye injuries treated in US emergency departments. Pediatrics. 2018;141(2):e20173083. https://doi.org/10.1542/peds.2017-3083.
22. Patel PA, Patel PN, Ahmed H. Epidemiologic trends in ophthalmic trauma related to major sports: an NEISS study. Ophthalmic Epidemiol. 2024;31(1):91–3.
23. U.S. Consumer Product Safety Commission, sports and recreational eye injuries, Washington: U.S. Consumer Product Safety Commission; 2000
24. Algarni AM, Guyatt GH, Turner A, Alamri S. Antibiotic prophylaxis for corneal abrasion. Cochrane Database Syst Rev. 2022;5(5):CD014617. Published 27 May 2022. https://doi.org/10.1002/14651858.CD014617.pub2.
25. Stephen C, Kaufman MD et al. Anterior segment trauma: evaluation, considerations and initial management. EyeWiki. https://eyewiki.aao.org/Anterior_Segment_Trauma:_Evaluation,_Considerations_and_Initial_Management. Published (if available).
26. Gudgel DT. Tips for prevention. Eye health tips & prevention. https://www.aao.org/eye-health/tips-prevention/injuries. Published 10 Apr 2023. Accessed 14 Oct 2023.
27. Gregory W, Oldham MD. Hyphema. EyeWiki. https://eyewiki.aao.org/Hyphema. Published 18 Oct 2023. Accessed 14 Oct 2023.
28. Stilger VG, Alt JM, Robinson TW. Traumatic hyphema in an intercollegiate baseball player: a case report. J Athl Train. 1999;34(1):25–8.
29. Walton W, Von Hagen S, Grigorian R, Zarbin M. Management of traumatic hyphema. Surv Ophthalmol. 2002;47(4):297–334. https://doi.org/10.1016/s0039-6257(02)00317-x.
30. Agrawal RV, Murthy S, Sangwan V, Biswas J. Current approach in diagnosis and management of anterior uveitis. Indian J Ophthalmol. 2010;58(1):11–9. https://doi.org/10.4103/0301-4738.58468.
31. Joseph Sowka OD, Alan GKOD. Develop a flare for uveitis. Review of optometry. https://www.reviewofoptometry.com/article/develop-a-flare-for-uveitis. Published 15 Jan 2006. Accessed 14 Oct 2023.
32. Walton RC. Traumatic uveitis. In: Ophthalmology in military and civilian casualty care. Springer International Publishing; 2019. p. 135.

33. Adedoyin Adesina MD. Corneal Laceration. eMedicine – Medscape. https://emedicine.medscape.com/article/798005-overview#a6. Accessed 14 Oct 2023.
34. Christopher R, Stelton MD, Mehul Rameshbhai Patel MD. Seidel test. EyeWiki. https://eyewiki.aao.org/Seidel_Test. Published 02 Aug 2023. Accessed 14 Oct 2023.
35. Hötte GJ, De Keizer ROB. Ocular injury and emergencies around the globe. Atlas Oral Maxillofac Surg Clin North Am. 2021;29(1):19–28. https://doi.org/10.1016/j.cxom.2020.11.002.
36. Porter D. What is corneal laceration. Eye health: diseases. https://www.aao.org/eye-health/diseases/what-is-corneal-laceration. Published 11 Oct 2022. Accessed 14 Oct 2023.
37. Kuhn F, Morris R, Witherspoon CD, Heimann K, Jeffers JB, Treister G. A standardized classification of ocular trauma. Ophthalmology. 1996;103(2):240–3. https://doi.org/10.1016/s0161-6420(96)30710-0.
38. Pieramici DJ. Open-globe injuries are rarely hopeless. Rev Ophthalmol. June 15, 2005. Accessed April 12, 2025. https://www.reviewofophthalmology.com/article/open-globe-injuries-are-rarely-hopeless
39. Kuhn F, Pelayes D. Management of the ruptured eye. Eur Ophthalmic Rev. 2009;3(1):48–50.
40. eyewiki.aao.org/Ruptured_Globe#cite_ref-kuhn17_14-0.
41. Fujikawa A, Mohamed YH, Kinoshita H, et al. Visual outcomes and prognostic factors in open-globe injuries. BMC Ophthalmol. 2018;18:138. https://doi.org/10.1186/s12886-018-0804-4.
42. Patel PA, Patel PN, Ahmed H. Epidemiologic trends in ophthalmic trauma related to major sports: an NEISS study. Ophthalmic epidemiology. 2024;31(1):91–3. https://doi.org/10.1080/09286586.2023.2173246. and (Cass SP. Ocular injuries in sports. Curr Sports Med Rep. 2012;11(1):1–15.
43. Nowlin B. Title of the Webpage. Society for American Baseball Research (SABR). https://sabr.org/bioproj/person/tony-conigliaro/. Accessed 14 Oct 2023.
44. Walton CR. Title of the Webpage. AJC.com. https://www.ajc.com/sports/baseball/timeline-the-baseball-helmet-history/39Ublld0jQO4OKPVUwddL/. Published 5 Oct 2009. Accessed 14 Oct 2023.
45. Newcomb T. The C-Flap continues its popular rise in MLB, Asian Markets. Baseball America. https://www.baseballamerica.com/stories/the-c-flap-continues-its-popular-rise-in-mlb-asian-markets/#:~:text=The%20flap%2C%20designed%20to%20attach,box%20following%20a%20face%20injury. Published 20 Mar 2019. Accessed 14 Oct 2023.
46. Marshall SW, Mueller FO, Kirby DP, Yang J. Evaluation of safety balls and faceguards for prevention of injuries in youth baseball. JAMA. 2003;289(5):568–74. https://doi.org/10.1001/jama.289.5.568.
47. Appearance of Little Leaguers in the Media. Little League. https://www.littleleague.org/downloads/appearance-little-leaguers-media/#:~:text=A%20face%20mask%20or%20face,approved%20(noted%20on%20helmet). Accessed 14 Oct 2023.
48. 1982–2020 NFHS risk minimization rules. National Federation of State High School Associations (NFHS). https://www.nfhs.org/media/4119363/1982-2020-nfhs-risk-minimization-rules-final-8-12-20.pdf. Accessed 14 Oct 2023.
49. New fast pitch rule for 2019–20 season. Mississippi High School Activities Association. https://www.misshsaa.com/2019/06/13/new-fast-pitch-rule-for-2019-20-season/. Accessed 14 Oct 2023.
50. Manual. Missouri State High School Activities Association. https://www.mshsaa.org/resources/Activities/Softball/Manual.pdf. Accessed 14 Oct 2023.
51. Softball mid-season updates & interpretations. Kentucky High School Athletic Association. https://khsaa.org/04-14-23-softball-mid-season-updates-interpretations/#:~:text=Since%202018%2C%20Kentucky%20has%20required,first%20basemen%2C%20and%20third%20basemen. Accessed 14 Oct 2023.
52. Danis RP, Hu K, Bell M. Acceptability of baseball face guards and reduction of oculofacial injury in receptive youth league players. Inj Prev. 2000;6(3):232–4. https://doi.org/10.1136/ip.6.3.232. Accessed 14 Oct 2023.

53. Higuchi T, Nagami T, Nakata H, Watanabe M, Isaka T, Kanosue K. Contribution of visual information about ball trajectory to baseball hitting accuracy. PLoS One. 2016;11(2):e0148498. Published 5 Feb 2016. https://doi.org/10.1371/journal.pone.0148498.
54. Palidis DJ, Wyder-Hodge PA, Fooken J, Spering M. Distinct eye movement patterns enhance dynamic visual acuity. PLoS One. 2017;12(2):e0172061. https://doi.org/10.1371/journal.pone.0172061. PMID: 28187157; PMCID: PMC5302791.
55. Uchida Y, Kudoh D, Higuchi T, Honda M, Kanosue K. Dynamic visual acuity in baseball players is due to superior tracking abilities. Med Sci Sports Exerc. 2013;45(2):319–25. https://doi.org/10.1249/MSS.0b013e31826fec97.
56. Laby DM, Rosenbaum AL, Kirschen DG, Davidson JL, Rosenbaum LJ, Strasser C, Mellman MF. The visual function of professional baseball players. Am J Ophthalmol. 1996;122(4):476–85. https://doi.org/10.1016/S0002-9394(14)72106-3.
57. Boghen D, Troost BT, Daroff RB, et al. Velocity characteristics of normal human saccades. Invest Ophthalmol. 1974;13:619–23.
58. Bahill AT, Brockenbrough A, Troost BT. Variability and development of a normative data base for saccadic eye movements. Invest Ophthalmol Vis Sci. 1981;21:116–25.
59. Bahill AT, LaRitz T. Why can't batters keep their eyes on the ball? Am Sci. 1984;72(3):249–53.
60. Meyer CH, Lasker AG, Robinson DA. The upper limit of human smooth pursuit velocity. Vision Res. 1985;25:561–3.
61. de Brouwer S, Yuksel D, Blohm G, et al. What triggers catch-up saccades during visual tracking? J Neurophysiol. 2002;87:1646–50.
62. Gray R, Cañal-Bruland R. Integrating visual trajectory and probabilistic information in baseball batting. Psychol Sport Exerc. 2018;36:123–31.
63. Kato T, Fukuda T. Visual search strategies of baseball batters: eye movements during the preparatory phase of batting. Percept Mot Skills. 2002;94(2):380–6. https://doi.org/10.2466/pms.2002.94.2.380.
64. Gray R, Regan D. Accuracy of estimating time to collision using binocular and monocular information. Vision Res. 1998;38:499–512.
65. Osborne K, Rudrud E, Zezoney F. Improved curveball hitting through the enhancement of visual cues. J Appl Behav Anal. 1990;23(3):371–7. https://doi.org/10.1901/jaba.1990.23-371.
66. Bahill AT, LaRitz T. Why can't batters keep their eyes on the ball? Am Sci. 1984;72:249–53.
67. Kishita Y, Ueda H, Kashino M. Eye and head movements of elite baseball players in real batting. Front Sports Act Living. 2020;2:3.
68. Laby DM. Sports vision. Focal Points American Academy of Ophthalmology. 2014;XXXII:1–15
69. Laby DM. Visual fixation in NBA free-throws and the relationship to on-court performance. Sports Perf Vis. 2020;2(1):1–7
70. Vickers JN. Mind over muscle: the role of gaze control, spatial cognition, and the quiet eye in motor expertise. Cogn Process. 2011;12(3):219–22. https://doi.org/10.1007/s10339-011-0411-2.
71. DeCouto B, Robertson CT, Lewis D, Mann DTY. The speed of perception: the effects of over-speed video training on pitch recognition in collegiate softball players. Cogn Process. 2020;21(1):77–93. https://doi.org/10.1007/s10339-019-00930-1.
72. Laby DM, Kirschen DG, Govindarajulu U, DeLand P. The effect of visual function on the batting performance of professional baseball players. Sci Rep. 2019;9(1):16847. Published 2019 Nov 14. https://doi.org/10.1038/s41598-019-52546-2.
73. Burris K, Vittetoe K, Ramger B, et al. Sensorimotor abilities predict on-field performance in professional baseball. Sci Rep. 2018;8(1):116. Published 2018 Jan 8. https://doi.org/10.1038/s41598-017-18565-7.
74. Laby DM, Kirschen DG, Govindarajulu U, DeLand P. The hand-eye coordination of professional baseball players: the relationship to batting. Optom Vis Sci. 2018;95(7):557–67. https://doi.org/10.1097/OPX.0000000000001239.

75. Classé JG, Semes LP, Daum KM, et al. Association between visual reaction time and batting, fielding, and earned run averages among players of the Southern Baseball League. J Am Optom Assoc. 1997;68(1):43–9.
76. Portal JM, Romano PE. Major review: ocular sighting dominance: a review and a study of athletic proficiency and eye-hand dominance in a collegiate baseball team. Binocul Vis Strabismus Q. 1998;13(2):125–32.
77. Laby DM, Kirschen DG. Thoughts on ocular dominance-is it actually a preference? Eye Contact Lens. 2011;37(3):140–4. https://doi.org/10.1097/ICL.0b013e31820e0bdf.
78. Laby DM, Appelbaum LG. Vision and on-field performance: a critical review of visual assessment and training studies with athletes. Optom Vis Sci. 2021;98(7):723–31. https://doi.org/10.1097/OPX.0000000000001729.
79. Khanal S. Impact of visual skills training on sports performance: current and future perspectives. MedCrave. 2015;2(1):1–3.
80. Maeda A, Komori Y, Shibayama H. Effects of training by using high speed pitched balls on kinetic visual acuity and bunt performance in baseball players. J Train Sci Exer Sport. 1999;11(1):1–8.
81. Kohmura Y, Yoshigi H. Training effects of visual function on college baseball players. HPM. 2004;1:15–23.
82. Deveau J, Ozer DJ, Seitz AR. Improved vision and on-field performance in baseball through perceptual learning. Curr Biol. 2014;24(4):R146–7. https://doi.org/10.1016/j.cub.2014.01.004.
83. Liu S, Ferris LM, Hilbig S, et al. Dynamic vision training transfers positively to batting performance among collegiate baseball batters. Psychol Sport Exerc. 2020;51:101759.
84. Laby D, Kirschen D. A new model for sports and performance vision. Vision Dev Rehabil. 2018;4(2):97–106.
85. Bowen T, Horth L. Use of the eyeport vision training system to enhance the visual performance of little league baseball players. JBO. 2005;16(6):143–8.

Chapter 4
Ophthalmology of Tennis

Ethan Waisberg, Joshua Ong, Mouayad Masalkhi, Miguel Crespo, and Andrew G. Lee

4.1 Introduction

Tennis requires a unique combination of stamina, hand-eye coordination, and agility. The International Tennis Federation estimates that over 106 million people play tennis across the world [1]. While the biomechanics of tennis are well understood, the underlying neuro-ophthalmic principles of the sport are rarely mentioned. The ability to quickly react and successfully return an up to 200 km/h

Author, Andrew G. Lee, MD, discloses that he has served or is serving as a consultant for the following companies: AstraZeneca, Alexion, Bristol Mayers Squibb, National Football League, Catalyst, Viridian, Ethyreal, NASA, US Department of Justice, Dompe, and Stoke.

E. Waisberg (✉)
Department of Clinical Neurosciences, University of Cambridge, Cambridge, UK
e-mail: ew690@cam.ac.uk

J. Ong
Department of Ophthalmology and Visual Sciences, University of Michigan Kellogg Eye Center, Ann Arbor, MI, USA

M. Masalkhi
University College Dublin School of Medicine, Belfield, Dublin, Ireland

M. Crespo
International Tennis Federation, London, UK

A. G. Lee
Department of Ophthalmology, Blanton Eye Institute, Houston Methodist Hospital, Houston, TX, USA

E. Waisberg et al. (eds.), *Ophthalmology of Sports*,
https://doi.org/10.1007/978-3-031-88645-4_4

serves is built upon various principles in neuro-ophthalmology. Although the average length of time per point is less than 10 s, these shorts bursts of plays require coordination between the eyes, brain, and extremities [2]. We aim to provide a resource for sports medicine providers, athletes, and ophthalmologists on the neuro-ophthalmic principles of tennis and how these fundamentals impact the game. These aspects include dynamic visual acuity, visual field, line-of-sight, saccade, and smooth pursuit. These principles may provide additional insight to athletes on the aspects that lead to proficient tennis playing and how improvements can be made in these areas.

4.2 Discussion

The key neuro-ophthalmic fundamentals of tennis include visual field, peripheral vision, static visual acuity, dynamic visual acuity, smooth pursuit, and saccades. We discuss these principles in relation to the game of tennis.

4.3 Static Visual Acuity (VA) and Dynamic Visual Acuity (DVA)

Tennis is played on a 78-foot-long, 27-foot-wide court during singles play and a 36-foot-wide court while playing doubles. Accurately visualizing a tennis ball and opponent from this distance requires a high level of baseline static visual acuity. This is essential at higher levels of tennis as the visual cues the opponent makes while hitting a shot (e.g., direction of swing and type of spin) are useful to know where this shot will be travelling. High levels of visual acuity are also necessary to make line calls. Both the line and landing point of the tennis ball must be sufficiently visualized to decisively make this call.

In the presence of bright sunlight that tennis is usually played in, visual acuity can be decreased due to glare. To reduce glare, some tennis players wear a brimmed hat and polarized sunglasses. Commercial sunglasses block up to 99–100% of the full ultraviolet spectrum [3]. These sunglasses should ideally be oversized or wraparound type to provide the most eye protection, by protecting against ultraviolet light entering from the sides of the eye. Plastic lenses would be most ideal for a tennis player, as it would be less likely to shatter on impact of a tennis ball.

Static visual acuity (SVA) refers to the ability to recognize characteristics of stationary objects whose images are formed on the retina when the examined subject remains still [4].

SVA can be affected by a variety of factors [4]. Contrast and brightness are two of the most important [4]. Other factors that affect SVA include age and refractive error [5]. If there is little contrast seen between a structure and its surroundings, the shape must be made bigger to be seen [4]. Furthermore, visual acuity steadily increases between 0.01 and 200 cd/cm^2, but this effect is limited as excessive light can produce glare and impair vision [4].

The measurement of a subject's static visual acuity has seen widespread use both as a screening tool in performance settings and for research into the underlying visual systems that support spatial vision [6]. One of the elements involved is the identification task, and it requires the participants to recognize a target similar to the one on the Snellen eye chart [6]. It is able to gauge letter identification, which is a requirement in everyday situations [6]. A resolution task is where subjects are required to differentiate a difference between the elements of a target (e.g., a grating pattern) [6].

Visual acuity is evaluated using the reciprocal of the visual angle in minutes of arc that is subtended at the eye by the smallest detail that can be detected [6]. One (1) is regarded as the standard score [6]. Landolt rings, cyclical gratings, and checkboards are all examples of tools that are frequently used for this task [6]. A detection task requires the participant to decide if a target exists or not, which also assesses the visual angle at which the target may be spotted. An acuity task asks participants to determine whether an upper vertical line is displaced to the right or the left of a lower line [6]. This allows the task to evaluate the visual angle of the smallest displacement that can be noticed by the subject [6].

Vernier acuity is utilized whenever there is a requirement to align two lines, such as when opening a combination lock or aligning a dial on a scale found in precision equipment [6]. A stereoscopic acuity task measures the ability to differentiate the different images received by the retinas of the two eyes of a single object that has depth [6]. This ability is measured by the difference between the parallactic images of two similar targets that are at just noticeably different distances from each other [6]. Stereoscopic acuity can be measured by a person's ability to differentiate the different images received by the retinas of the two eyes of a single object that has depth [6]. This aspect of neuro-ophthalmology in tennis has been investigated. Kutzner et al. observed that tennis players consisting of professions, former professionals, and coaches completed dynamic stereoscopic tasks, and their stereoscopic performance improved which include response time and stereo acuity [7].

Giblin et al. [8] examined the influence of visual occlusion on the tennis serve, by examining players serving with their eyes open and closed. The visual occlusion led to players being unable to make contact on 16 of 24 serves and caused alterations in both ball and racket kinematics. This study shows that visual feedback is crucial for the spaciotemporal regulation of a tennis serve.

4.4 Dynamic Visual Acuity

Dynamic visual acuity (DVA) refers to the ability to visualize an object while in motion [9, 10]. High levels of DVA are essential as a tennis player while tracking the constantly moving ball, particularly during the return of serve which can be over 120mph. The tennis ball remains in constant motion throughout an entire point. The ability to track a tennis ball constantly throughout a match requires high levels of DVA.

The capacity to see fine details even when there is movements between an observer and the item being observed is known as DVA [11]. When the eyes cannot catch up to the speed of a moving pattern, component of the pattern might not be consistently captured on the fovea [12]. It was found that when the velocity of target motion approached roughly 60° per second, DVA began to decline significantly [13].

4.5 Visual Anticipation

Visual anticipation in tennis involves using visual cues to anticipate an opponent's intended actions and is a key component of elite tennis performance. Professional tennis players routinely anticipate the location of an opponent's serve, when behind the baseline or at the net. Visual anticipation involves both non-kinematic (e.g., opponent's court positioning) and kinematic visual cues. An analysis of ball trajectory recordings from singles matches of professional players found that the probability of hitting a cross-court shot increased significantly when the player was positioned close to the single's sideline [14]. This shot is most intuitive for tennis players to hit in this position, as a cross-court shot passes over the center of the net (lowest net height) and allows the player to have a greater depth error tolerance.

Shim et al. [15] examined which sources of visual information are used by highly skilled tennis players as anticipatory cues of the direction of an opponent's shots. This study found that while different types of shots can be anticipated, the direction of the shot is more difficult to anticipate. An additional finding of this study was that occlusion of the forearm and racket significantly decreased the ability of a participant to determine the type of stroke produced.

4.6 Visual Field

The ability in tennis to be able to see your opponent in your peripheral vision, while still primarily looking at the tennis ball is crucial. Tennis players are required to look at the tennis ball prior to and even during the point of impact, to ensure the ball is hit near the center of the racket. While still making contact with the ball, elite tennis players are using their peripheral vision to see the location of their opponent and are able to hit the ball away from this location. Strong peripheral vision can also be crucial for making no-look shots, which adds another layer of deception against the opponent.

The field of vision is the region of space that may be observed simultaneously while focused in one direction [16]. The monocular visual field is split into two sections: central vision, which comprises the center of fixation and the inner 30° of vision, and peripheral vision, which encompasses the outer 100°, middle 60°, upper 60°, and lower 75° [16]. Visual field testing can be performed in a variety of methods, including automated static perimetry, Goldmann kinetic perimetry, and confrontation testing at the patient's bedside [16].

The line of sight (LOS) is the path of the beam from the fixation point via the pupil center (PC) and into the foveola [16]. The LOS represents the diverted beam of light that goes via each optical interface on its journey from the fixation point to the PC and finally, after refraction, to the foveola [16]. When compared to the visual axis, the LOS is linked with a much longer optical path difference (OPD) [16]. To estimate LOS, two light sources positioned at different distances from the eye can be utilized simultaneously—one focused on the retina and the other out of focus [16]. If the primary rays from both sources overlap and land on the LOS, the ray from the out-of-focus source will generate a fuzzy circle, while the beam from the focused source will make the center of the blur circle [16].

4.7 Color Vision

In 1972, the International Tennis Federation introduced the switch from white or black tennis balls to neon yellow tennis ball to maximize visibility to viewers watching on television [17]. In a similar capacity for players on the court, having adequate color vision may be helpful in tennis to visualize the ball moving at high speeds. Color vision is the capacity to distinguish between photons with different spectral compositions, independent of intensity [18]. Color vision is based on evaluating information from photoreceptors with varying levels of spectral sensitivities [18].

Humans with normal color vision can discern hundreds of colors [18]. To accomplish this, we use signals from three different types of cone photoreceptors, whose strongest sensitivity ranges from short (S, 430 nm), medium (M, 530 nm), and long (L, 560 nm) wavelengths, but whose tuning is broad enough that each reacts to light across most of the visible spectrum, resulting in "trichromatic" human vision [18]. The spectrum sensitivity of a mammalian photoreceptor is determined by the opsin it generates, which is covalently connected to a chromophore in the outer segment [18]. The arrangement of amino acids in the opsin protein defines its spectrum sensitivity, and any changes in its sequence can have a significant influence on its function [18].

4.8 Saccades vs Smooth Pursuit

During a tennis match, there are a variety of competing visual stimuli, and visual attention must be directed at the most important sources of information. Saccades are brief, quick eye movements that allow the observer to notice an item in the visual field and concentrate it on the fovea, boosting the potential for discernment [19]. The relative saccade direction is determined by comparing the absolute saccade trajectories of two successive saccades [19]. To provide discretized saccade directions, the absolute saccade direction is grouped into predefined angular segments [19]. Complex neural signals in the Superior Colliculus (SC) and Frontal Eye Field (FEF) are essential for saccade preparation, with the former being linked to the pupil control circuit [19].

A saccadic eye movement to orient to the thing being sought is usually followed by a regular smooth pursuit movement [19]. The pursuit mechanism then matches the eye's motion with the velocity of the item [19]. This movement is stopped by saccadic eye movements that decrease retinal error between the present gaze location and the target [19]. Smooth pursuit has a delay of 100–125 ms compared to 200–250 ms for saccades [20, 21].

Rosker et al. [22] examined the correlations between gaze fixations and areas of interest during tennis serve return in 10 national and 5 international level tennis players. Focal visual attention was measured with an eye movement tracking device and 675 returns of serve were analyzed. This study found that the national level players exhibited less specific gaze behavior than the international level players and that international level players had additional gaze behavior during the follow through phase to increase performance.

Lafont [23] examined the gaze position during the hitting phase of a tennis stroke. This study used over 5000 high-resolution photos of groundstrokes of players ranked in the top 100 in the Association of Tennis Professionals (ATP) and Women Tennis Association (WTA), and these photos were analyzed by three tennis experts. This study found that elite tennis players have a head fixation at the point of impact while making contact with a tennis ball and during the follow-through, while near elite tennis players do not share this same fixation pattern.

4.9 Ocular Trauma

While relatively rare, ocular trauma in tennis can cause permanent visual damage. In 1912, William Laurentz, a top ranked French tennis player, had a tennis ball glance him in the eye following contact with the side of his racket, which subsequently required removal of his eye [24]. Despite this eye removal, he continued to perform at a high level and represented France in Davis Cup tennis.

Seelenfreund et al. [25] reported a series of ten patients sustaining ocular contusion injuries secondary to the blunt force trauma from a tennis ball. Seven of the ten patients in this study required laser photocoagulation, retinal surgery, or both [25]. This study shows the potential ophthalmic risks of tennis, particularly when volleying close to the net and advises that eye protection be worn in certain high-risk individuals.

Patel et al. [26] conducted a retrospective observational study of the National Electronic Injury Surveillance System to examine eye injuries related to tennis in the United States over a 20-year period. Approximately 16,000 tennis-related eye injuries were identified, and males were nearly two times more likely to be affected [26]. The spring season had the greatest proportion of injury occurrence. The age group with the greatest proportion of injuries was boys aged 11–15 years. Although the majority of these patients did not have serious visual consequences, the risk of amblyopia is high in this age group.

4.10 Blind Tennis

Although this chapter highlights the importance of visual function for tennis, this is not always a requirement to play the sport. Blind tennis is a sport first developed in Japan in 1984, by a blind individual wishing to play tennis [27]. Blind tennis uses special tennis balls, which make a distinctive noise when it is bounced or hit [27]. This allows a player to respond to auditory cues rather than visual cues to understand when to hit a ball. These tennis balls also travel slower and are lighter, making them easier to hit. Shorter and lighter tennis rackets are also used, making them easier to maneuver. Rather than visualizing the boundary lines on the court, the blind players use tactile sensation and touch the lines to determine their court positioning [27]. Blind tennis allows a blind person to not only play a great sport and have physical activity, but to also further develop further independence, spatial awareness skills, physical coordination, and social skills.

4.11 Conclusion

The key neuro-ophthalmic fundamentals of tennis include visual field, static visual acuity, dynamic visual acuity, saccades, smooth pursuit, and color vision. These fundamental aspects of neuro-ophthalmology play a critical role in the proficiency of tennis [7]. Future work is necessary to develop a standardized vocabulary for defining the precise role of these neuro-ophthalmic principles in tennis. Future work is also required on how visual status and vision deficits can impact tennis performance [28, 29].

Author Contributions Ethan Waisberg – Design, Writing

Joshua Ong – Design, Writing
Mouayad Masalkhi – Writing, Review
Miguel Crespo – Review, Intellectual Support
Andrew G. Lee – Review, Intellectual Support

Disclosures Dr. Andrew G. Lee is a consultant for the National Football League (NFL), NASA, and the US Department of Justice (DOJ). Dr. Lee is a consultant for Amgen/Horizon, AstraZeneca, Alexion, Viridian, Dompe, Catalyst, Ethyreal, Stoke, and Bristol Myers Squibb.

References

1. ITF global tennis report- 2024. International Tennis Federation. London.
2. Kovacs MS. Tennis physiology: training the competitive athlete. Sports Med. 2007;37(3):189–98. https://doi.org/10.2165/00007256-200737030-00001.
3. How to pick the best sunglasses to protect your eyes. Published 8 July 2019. Accessed 31 Dec 2022. How to pick the best sunglasses to protect your eyes.
4. Rabbetts RB. Bennett & Rabbetts' clinical visual optics. 4th ed. Elsevier/Butterworth Heinemann; 2007.
5. Eames TH. Correspondence between visual acuity, refractive error, and the speed of visual perception. Br J Ophthalmol. 1953;37(5):312–3. https://doi.org/10.1136/bjo.37.5.312.
6. Chan AHS, Courtney AJ. Foveal acuity, peripheral acuity and search performance: a review. Int J Ind Ergon. 1996;18(2):113–9. https://doi.org/10.1016/0169-8141(95)00073-9.
7. Kutzner BL, Ring M, Michelson G. Binokulares Sehtraining bei Hochleistungssportlern. Fortschr Ophthalmol. 2022;119(7):721–9. https://doi.org/10.1007/s00347-022-01574-x.
8. Giblin G, Whiteside D, Reid M. Now you see, now you don't … the influence of visual occlusion on racket and ball kinematics in the tennis serve. Sports Biomech. 2017;16(1):23–33. https://doi.org/10.1080/14763141.2016.1179337.
9. Waisberg E, Ong J, Zaman N, Kamran SA, Lee AG, Tavakkoli A. Head-mounted dynamic visual acuity for G-transition effects during interplanetary spaceflight: technology development and results from an early validation study. Aerosp Med Hum Perform. 2022;93(11):800–5. https://doi.org/10.3357/AMHP.6092.2022.
10. Waisberg E, Ong J, Paladugu P, et al. Dynamic visual acuity as a biometric for astronaut performance and safety. Life Sci Space Res. 2023;37:3–6. https://doi.org/10.1016/j.lssr.2023.01.002.
11. Waisberg E, Ong J, Zaman N, Kamran SA, Lee AG, Tavakkoli A. Stroboscopic augmented reality as an approach to mitigate gravitational transition effects during interplanetary spaceflight. Int J Aviat Aeronaut Aerosp. 2022;9(4):6. https://commons.erau.edu/ijaaa
12. Murphy BJ. Pattern thresholds for moving and stationary gratings during smooth eye movement. Vis Res. 1978;18(5):521–30. https://doi.org/10.1016/0042-6989(78)90196-7.
13. Burg A. Visual acuity as measured by dynamic and static tests: a comparative evaluation. J Appl Psychol. 1966;50:460–6. https://doi.org/10.1037/h0023982.
14. Huesmann K, Loffing F. Contextual cue utilization in visual anticipation in tennis: on the role of an opponent's on-court position and skill. Ger J Exerc Sport Res. 2019;49(3):304–12. https://doi.org/10.1007/s12662-019-00597-y.
15. Shim J, Miller G, Lutz R. Visual cues and information used to anticipate tennis ball shot and placement. J Sport Behav. 2005;28(2):186–200.
16. Mosquera SA, Verma S, McAlinden C. Centration axis in refractive surgery. Eye Vis (Lond). 2015;2:4. https://doi.org/10.1186/s40662-015-0014-6.

17. History of tennis balls. Published November 2019. Accessed 14 Jan 2023. https://www.itftennis.com/media/2280/balls-history-of-tennis-balls.pdf.
18. Solomon SG, Lennie P. The machinery of colour vision. Nat Rev Neurosci. 2007;8(4):276–86. https://doi.org/10.1038/nrn2094.
19. Mahanama B, Jayawardana Y, Rengarajan S, et al. Eye movement and pupil measures: a review. Front Comput Sci. 2022;3:733531. Accessed 27 Dec 2022. https://www.frontiersin.org/articles/10.3389/fcomp.2021.733531.
20. Meyer CH, Lasker AG, Robinson DA. The upper limit of human smooth pursuit velocity. Vis Res. 1985;25(4):561–3. https://doi.org/10.1016/0042-6989(85)90160-9.
21. Krauzlis RJ. Recasting the smooth pursuit eye movement system. J Neurophysiol. 2004;91(2):591–603. https://doi.org/10.1152/jn.00801.2003.
22. Rosker J, Majcen RZ. Correlations between gaze fixations to different areas of interest are related to tennis serve return performance in two different expert groups. Int J Perform Anal Sport. 2021;21(6):1149–61. https://doi.org/10.1080/24748668.2021.1979840.
23. Lafont D. Gaze control during the hitting phase in tennis: a preliminary study. Int J Perform Anal Sport. 2008;8(1):85–100. https://doi.org/10.1080/24748668.2008.11868425.
24. Duke M. Tennis players and eye injuries. JAMA. 1976;236(20):2287. https://doi.org/10.1001/jama.1976.03270210019010.
25. Seelenfreund MH. Rushing the net and retinal detachment. JAMA. 1976;235(25):2723. https://doi.org/10.1001/jama.1976.03260510017016.
26. Patel PS, Uppuluri A, Oydanich M, Langer PD, Zarbin MA, Bhagat N. Epidemiology of United States tennis-related ocular injuries from 2000 to 2019. Int Ophthalmol. Published online September. 2022;43:997–1003. https://doi.org/10.1007/s10792-022-02502-3.
27. Matsui A. Blind tennis manual. Tennis Ireland. Published 2014. Accessed 2 Jan 2023. https://www.tennisireland.ie/wp-content/uploads/2016/10/4.-Blind-Tennis-Coaching-Manual.pdf.
28. Waisberg E, Ong J, Paladugu P, et al. Optimizing screening for preventable blindness with head-mounted visual assessment technology. J Visual Impair Blin. 2022;116(4):579–81. https://doi.org/10.1177/0145482X221124186.
29. Waisberg E, Ong J, Paladugu P, et al. Advances in machine learning to detect preventable causes of blindness. Eye. Published online December. 2022;10:2582. https://doi.org/10.1038/s41433-022-02354-2.

Chapter 5
Sports Ophthalmology: Soccer

Alex Suh, Andrew Suh, Gilad Hampel, Joshua Ong, Matthew Lam, Jose Comenarez Moreno, Linxia Gu, and Donny Suh

5.1 Introduction

Soccer, more popularly known as football worldwide, (in distinction to the entirely different sport of "American football" in the United States) has a historical footprint stretching back to ancient civilizations [1]. Through several adaptations and modifications, the sport has evolved into the most popular and widely played game worldwide. The establishment of international organizations such as the Football Association in England in 1863 and the inaugural Federation Internationale de Football Association (FIFA) World Cup in 1930 have sculpted the sport's adoration and global recognition. Even already the most popular sport, participation in soccer has grown tremendously over the last three decades in the United States [2]. The high-intensity and direct contact with consistent changes in movement, velocity, and direction provide immense entertainment as well as potential risks. Although the most popular sport, it causes a disproportionate number of eye injuries in individuals under the age of 25 years old [3].

A. Suh (✉) · A. Suh · G. Hampel
Tulane University School of Medicine, New Orleans, LA, USA
e-mail: asuh@tulane.edu

J. Ong
Department of Ophthalmology and Visual Sciences, University of Michigan Kellogg Eye Center, Ann Arbor, MI, USA

M. Lam
University of Colorado School of Medicine, Aurora, CO, USA

J. C. Moreno · L. Gu
Department of Biomedical and Mechanical Engineering, Florida Institute of Technology, Melbourne, FL, USA

D. Suh
University of California Irvine School of Medicine, Irvine, CA, USA

E. Waisberg et al. (eds.), *Ophthalmology of Sports*,
https://doi.org/10.1007/978-3-031-88645-4_5

Furthermore, ocular trauma is significant in the pediatric population as more than half of all sports-related eye injuries are in patients ≤18 years of age [4]. This is partly because the sport requires the least amount of equipment (e.g., protective eyewear) compared to other sports, adding to its simplicity [5].

In parallel to soccer's soaring popularity, considering the potential risks and safety concerns must be further evaluated within the sport. Ocular trauma, in particular, poses a significant concern for players, due to the sport's inherent physical contact, quick pace, and use of a solid ball. Injuries may arise from elbows to the face, stray fingers to the eyes, and even forceful impacts from the ball. Minor superficial abrasions to more severe outcomes such as orbital fracture and eyelid lacerations may arise from the fast-paced sport [3]. Implications of ocular trauma can impact the player's vision and performance and can even extend beyond the field. Recognizing the significance of ocular safety may provide further insight on the need for preventative measures and protective equipment [6]. Safety guidelines, referee vigilance, and possibly protective eyewear may all be expounded upon to reduce the risk of eye injuries. This chapter aims to provide a deeper understanding of ocular trauma in the sport of soccer and provide insight on potential strategies to enhance player safety, promote awareness, and minimize the occurrence of preventable injuries.

5.2 Rules of Soccer

The game of soccer includes two teams, two goals, and one soccer ball. Each team contains 11 players with a total of 22 players on the field at one time. Among the 11 players on each team, there is usually one goalie, four defenders, three midfielders, and three forwards. However, different formations are used by different teams to play to their strengths. Defenders are players who play near their own goal defending from the other team, preventing them from scoring. Midfield players are involved in both the defense and offense of their team, preventing the opponents from scoring while also trying to score on the opponent's goal. Forwards are players who are focused on offense trying to score on the opposing team. The soccer goals are placed on opposite sides of the field, and the objective of the game is to score more goals than the opposing team. A rectangular field is used with specific measurements on how large the field and different boundaries are as seen in Fig. 5.1 [7]. Of note, there have been no major changes to the rules of soccer sufficient enough to affect player safety in recent years. This indicates that much of the research cited in this chapter is still of relevance.

The main rules of soccer are that any part of the body can be used to control the soccer ball except the hands and arms of a player. Soccer games have two 45 min halves with stoppage time added at the end of each half. Like many other sports, there are penalty kicks and fouls when players are too aggressive or break rules of the game, such as using their hands in play. Whichever team the ball touches last before going out of the lines of the field, the opposite team obtains possession. The soccer ball can be put back into play by goal kicks, corner kicks, or throw-ins. Whichever team has more goals scored by the end of the second half plus stoppage time is the winner of the match.

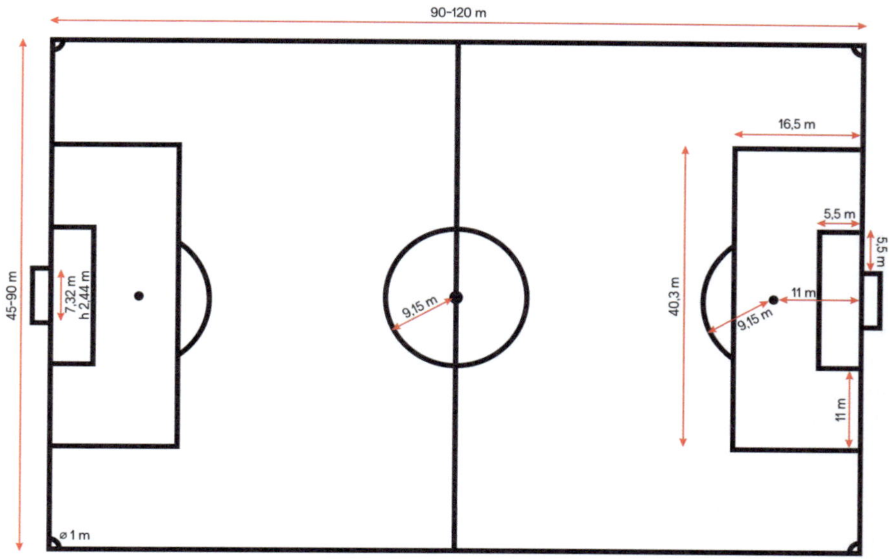

Fig. 5.1 Dimensions of a standard soccer field. Reprinted with permission under the Creative Commons License. For more details, visit Creative Commons Attribution 4.0 International License (https://creativecommons.org/licenses/by/4.0/). The diagram provides precise measurements and layout specifications for a standard soccer field, aiding in understanding the field's geometry for sports analysis and design applications

5.3 Ocular Trauma in Soccer

In a 2016 study, 2054 soccer-related facial trauma entries from the National Electronic Injury Surveillance System (NEISS) were analyzed, which consisted of lacerations, contusions, and fractures. The nose was the most common fracture site (75.1%), most commonly occurring due to head-to-head collisions (39.0%). Pediatric patients (<19 years of age) accounted for approximately 67% of injuries, whereas adult male athletes were at the highest risk of fractures [8]. Yang et al. (2019) reported that these encounters often occur during boys' soccer competitions when players were chasing a loose ball and collided [9]. Although soccer tends to have less ocular-related trauma relative to other sports (e.g., basketball, baseball, football), the sport has been significantly associated with more "major" anterior and posterior ocular injuries [10].

The incidence of eye injury in any single soccer game may be small, but the vast popularity of the sport worldwide poses a problem for society [6]. One study found that indoor soccer injuries are the most prevalent at 50.9%, followed by outdoor soccer at 47.2%, with the rest being beach, volleyball, and intramural soccer [3]. Most injuries were due to direct impacts or rebounds by the ball (79.1%), while 6.1% were due to fists and 6.1% due to foot traumas. Most injuries (95.1%) were considered to be accidental. Filipe et al. also assessed the areas of highest injury probability; 60.1% of injuries occurred near the goalpost, whereas 34.4% occurred near the midfield. Furthermore, forwards comprised 38.7% of the on-field injuries, and defenders comprised 30.7%. Additionally, ocular injuries in soccer most commonly occur in adolescent athletes [11].

One of the most prevalent types of ocular injury in soccer is blunt trauma to the eye (e.g., balls, elbows, accidental collisions with other players). Severe cases of traumatic macular holes, retinal detachment, retinal tears and hemorrhage, choroidal rupture, and vitreous hemorrhage and Berlin's edema have been studied in the past [13]. One study found that simply heading the ball cannot create enough energy to cause retinal hemorrhages, but a direct impact to the eye can cause a retinal tear or injury [14]. During a direct soccer ball impact to the eye, high intraocular pressure and stress can manifest from direct transmission of force from the ball. These pressures can propagate as a wave of compressive and tractional forces on the retina, subsequently inducing retinal hemorrhaging [15]. The sudden compression and decompression impulse within the eyeball from impact can also induce retinal tears and detachments due to the delicate nature of the tissue. A forceful encounter with a soccer ball to the ocular orbit is spread out over a period of 10 ms, which is relatively longer compared to other sports balls (e.g., golf, baseball). The impact may be shallower, but the prolonged presence in the orbital space also provides profound opportunity for damage [6]. Felipe et al. further addressed the mechanism behind a soccer ball's ability to cause ocular injury despite the size discrepancy between the ball and the orbit [12]. The ball deforms on impact enough to have a "…small 'knuckle' of the ball… enter the orbit and impact the globe." [12] Furthermore, a secondary suction effect produced further injury on the orbit. However, they found that ball air pressure did not significantly change ball penetration.

The cornea, being the outermost protective layer of the eye, can experience abrasions or lacerations due to the sheer force of the impact. A forceful collision may also lead to lens dislocation. Corneal abrasions were found to be the most common type of ocular injury in soccer along with hyphema and vitreous hemorrhages [16]. Corneal foreign bodies are also potential injuries during gameplay. Lacerations, perforation, rupture, mucocutaneous, and nervous injuries are all other possibilities. Ultimately, when assessing ocular injury in a post-game ophthalmologic setting, a comprehensive ophthalmologic exam should be done to rule out any and all types of ophthalmologic injury.

5.4 Management and Prevention of Ocular Trauma in Soccer

Ocular trauma has been a prevalent problem in all sports, but especially soccer due to the eyes being an extremely vulnerable site to injury. Unlike many other sports at the professional level (e.g., American football, baseball, lacrosse, and hockey) that require protective equipment like helmets and pads, soccer does not require any protective equipment besides shin guards [7]. In recent years, protective eyewear has been introduced towards the sports community to help solve and limit the severity of eye injuries in sports. It has been determined from previous research that protective eyewear can lower the risk of significant eye injury by more than 90% [17, 18]. Analyzing and advocating for protective eyewear is pivotal to prevent ocular trauma in young athletes and recreational players [3].

Research analyzing the efficacy of protective eyewear during soccer-induced ocular trauma has demonstrated it is a strong method of reducing injury-inducing retinal stress [5]. Nowadays, protective eyewear is constructed of either polycarbonate or acrylic material. However, there is a debate on which material is optimal for the most protection given all circumstances. In a 2023 study, protective eyewear made out of polycarbonate and acrylic material was compared in the reduction of retinal strain and stress experienced by the eye. In the experiment, the polycarbonate material outperformed the protective eyewear made out of acrylic for both the retinal stress and strain experienced by the eye, signifying polycarbonate as the optimal medium for protective eyewear [5]. However, both the polycarbonate and acrylic models reduced the severity of deformations of the eye compared to the unprotected eye model, suggesting protective eyewear will reduce the severity of ocular trauma regardless of material.

Protective eyewear has been recommended for patients who have prescription lenses, one eye, or for those who have had refractive surgical procedures that weaken the eye [12]. However, protective eyewear needs to be advocated for healthy athletes to prevent detrimental and irreversible ocular trauma. The evidence supporting the efficacy of protective eyewear emphasizes the pressing needs for increased awareness and advocacy within the sports community, helping to preserve the ocular health among athletes. Prevention and management of ocular injuries should begin early with on-field recognition and care administration. It has been recommended to train soccer athletes with skills to identify hazards and develop quick responses to avoiding injury-risk behaviors [19]. Training players early to predict behaviors that could result in ocular injury could help mitigate high-risk situations. Teaching players a sense of "awareness" of an oncoming collision is a strategy associated with a decreased injury severity and recovery times [20]. Such high-risk situations include aerial duels (e.g., during corner kicks, free kicks), which pose a risk for head-to-head collisions or problematic landings. Engaging in rough play and aggressive challenges with opponents may also lead to high-risk tackles, so emotional awareness and active practice of sportsmanship is also a critical component of instruction. Coaching players to recognize these situations early could be a first step in "preventative medicine" to reduce ocular injuries in soccer. Additionally, training players to recognize ocular injury early could allow them to start providing care immediately on the field before healthcare personnel even have the opportunity to intervene. For example, players could recognize the symptoms of a corneal foreign body, and they could prevent the player from rubbing their eye and causing further abrasion.

Contact lenses in comparison to spectacles provide no additional protection against eye impact or corneal injury and may even pose a risk to contributing additional corneal abrasion or corneal laceration with rupture of the eye. Eyeglasses however also pose a risk to shattering during impact, especially if they do not meet eye protection standards. For example, a report on badminton players found penetrating ocular injuries due to shattered glass spectacles [22]. Therefore, other solutions (e.g., face masks) may provide an alternative solution to eye protection without the danger of shattering. If players do utilize eyewear, they should meet sports eyewear ASTM F803 standards outlined by Vinger et al. [21]

5.5 Vision-Related Considerations

Soccer is a highly dynamic and visually demanding sport, thereby placing a significant reliance on a player's visual abilities. Ball control, decision-making, spatial awareness, and overall performance require optimal vision. As the most essential sense in sports, vision and visual queues are vital to soccer gameplay [23]. Depth perception is possibly the most important aspect required, since it is necessary for a player to judge ball trajectory, goal, and distance. Furthermore, ball handling relies on visual inputs and proprioceptive inputs from the limbs to accurately move the ball as intended. Peripheral vision is also vital to playmaking, since players must be aware of their surroundings to assess opposing players' attacking or teammates for potential passes. Ongoing research in neuro-ophthalmology and even vision training programs develop new insights in the assessment and optimization of player performance and safety.

Burris et al. (2019) researched the visual, perceptual, and motor skills of several high-achieving athletes. They found that strategic sports (e.g., soccer) require players to maintain an array of visual information about teammates, opponents, and the ball. Players with higher abilities in Perception Span were able to quickly code and preserve spatial information, thus performing better with skills such as pattern recognition and recall, decision-making, and team mental model development [24]. Knollner et al. (2022) explored deeper specifically in elite soccer players and found a relationship between visual skills and executive functions [25]. One potential idea for this relationship is that more efficient neuronal processing of visual input provides greater resources for cognitive processing [26]. Essentially, elite soccer players may be able to process visual information more efficiently so that they free up space for processing strategy, pattern recognition, and teamwork on the field. Near-Far Quickness is described as one's ability to quickly switch focus between objects of differing distances [27]. This ability, as well as hand-eye coordination, has been linked to stronger executive function, possibly due to greater cognitive flexibility and the attentional control-subcomponent of the working memory system [28]. This suggests that a stronger visual system lays a foundation for performance enhancements of executive functions [25].

If performance is truly enhanced by visual skills, then training visual skills may potentially translate over to an increased sports performance. Formenti et al. (2019) conducted a 6-week vision training session on female volleyball players and demonstrated an increase in cognitive functions. The vision training sport-specific group also tended to have enhanced clinical reaction time, which suggests that vision training may be a valid modality for increased performance. However, Theofilou et al. (2022) conducted a similar experiment on soccer players and found no further benefits to reaction time, physical fitness, and cognitive function compared to the traditional soccer training program [29]. Evidently, future studies are warranted to further explore the potential effects of visual stimuli training programs on sports performance. In the advent of rapidly developing virtual and augmented reality software and hardware, vision training may become integrated into the elite athlete programs of the future.

5.6 Summary

Despite immense popularity, the high-speed and intense nature of soccer poses inherent risks to the eye. This chapter delved into the types of injuries, etiologies, and potential consequences of ocular trauma in soccer. With the high prevalence and increase in popularity of the sport, it is evermore important to consider the importance of eye protection during competition. The significance of early recognition of high-risk situations is paramount as educating players on potential hazards (e.g., aerial duels, aggressive behavior) may lead to a reduction in injury occurrences. With soccer being the most popular sport in the world and its growing popularity in the United States, it is pivotal to acknowledge the danger of ocular injury.

The ongoing development of vision training programs and virtual reality technologies hint at future possibilities in improving not only player performance but also visual and cognitive skills. Protective eyewear is perhaps the most critical method in reducing the probability of blunt eye injury, with past research suggesting polycarbonate as the best medium for protective eyewear. Additionally, raising awareness of ocular injuries among players and coaches could help reduce the incidence by preventing them on the field. While celebrating its dynamic environment and global appeal, it is equally essential to address the potential risks it poses. Fostering a culture of ocular awareness, education, and injury prevention can ensure that soccer continues to captivate the world while securing the well-being and safety of its players.

References

1. Soccer is the world's most popular sport. But who invented it?. National Geographic. Published June 8, 2023. Accessed 13 Aug 2023.
2. Giulianotti R, Robertson R. Globalization and football. Sage; 2009.
3. Capao Filipe JA, Fernandes VL, Barros H, Falcao-Reis F, Castro-Correia J. Soccer-related ocular injuries. Arch Ophthalmol Chic Ill 1960. 2003;121(5):687–94. https://doi.org/10.1001/archopht.121.5.687.

4. Haring RS, Sheffield ID, Canner JK, Schneider EB. Epidemiology of sports-related eye injuries in the United States. JAMA Ophthalmol. 2016;134(12):1382–90. https://doi.org/10.1001/jamaophthalmol.2016.4253.
5. Suh A, Lam M, Shokrollahi Y, Dong P, Gu L, Suh D. Quantifying the efficacy of protective eyewear in pediatric soccer-induced retinal injury. J AAPOS Off Publ Am Assoc Pediatr Ophthalmol Strabismus. 2023;27(3):131.e1–6. https://doi.org/10.1016/j.jaapos.2023.02.009.
6. Vinger PF, Capão Filipe JA. The mechanism and prevention of soccer eye injuries. Br J Ophthalmol. 2004;88(2):167–8. https://doi.org/10.1136/bjo.2003.026229.
7. The International Football Association Board (IFAB). Laws of the Game 22/23. Published online July 1, 2022.
8. Bobian MR, Hanba CJ, Svider PF, et al. Soccer-related facial trauma: a nationwide perspective. Ann Otol Rhinol Laryngol. 2016;125(12):992–6. https://doi.org/10.1177/0003489416668195.
9. Yang Y, Liller K, Morris B, Fillion J, Bubu O. Injuries among young Florida athletes playing sports in recreational leagues. Fla Public Health Rev. 2019;14(1):13. https://digitalcommons.unf.edu/fphr/vol14/iss1/13
10. Patel V, Pakravan P, Mehra D, Watane A, Yannuzzi NA, Sridhar J. Trends in sports-related ocular trauma in United States emergency departments from 2010 to 2019: multi-center cross-sectional study. Semin Ophthalmol. 2023;38(4):333–7. https://doi.org/10.1080/08820538.2022.2107400.
11. Burke MJ, Sanitato JJ, Vinger PF, Raymond LA, Kulwin DR. Soccerball-induced eye injuries. JAMA. 1983;249(19):2682–5.
12. Capão Filipe JA. Soccer (football) ocular injuries: an important eye health problem. Br J Ophthalmol. 2004;88(2):159–60. https://doi.org/10.1136/bjo.2003.031518.
13. Horn EP, McDonald HR, Johnson RN, et al. Soccer ball-related retinal injuries: a report of 13 cases. Retina Phila Pa. 2000;20(6):604–9. https://doi.org/10.1097/00006982-200011000-00003.
14. Reed WF, Feldman KW, Weiss AH, Tencer AF. Does soccer ball heading cause retinal bleeding? Arch Pediatr Adolesc Med. 2002;156(4):337–40. https://doi.org/10.1001/archpedi.156.4.337.
15. Lam MR, Dong P, Shokrollahi Y, Gu L, Suh DW. Finite element analysis of soccer ball-related ocular and retinal trauma and comparison with abusive head trauma. Ophthalmol Sci. 2022;2(2):100129. https://doi.org/10.1016/j.xops.2022.100129.
16. Tucker AM. Common soccer injuries: diagnosis, treatment and rehabilitation. Sports Med. 1997;23:21–32.
17. Gledhill A, Forsdyke D. An ounce of prevention is better than a pound of cure: shouldn't we be doing EVERYTHING to reduce sports injury incidence and burden? Br J Sports Med. 2018;52(20):1292–3. https://doi.org/10.1136/bjsports-2018-099208.
18. Mishra A, Verma AK. Sports related ocular injuries. Med J Armed Forces India. 2012;68(3):260–6. https://doi.org/10.1016/j.mjafi.2011.12.004.
19. Zuckerman S, Totten D, Rubel K, et al. 174 mechanisms of injury as a diagnostic predictor of sport-related concussion severity in football, basketball, and soccer: results from a regional concussion registry. Neurosurgery. 2016;63:102–12. https://doi.org/10.1227/01.neu.0000489743.00212.e6.
20. Wasserman EB, Kerr ZY, Zuckerman SL, Covassin T. Epidemiology of sports-related concussions in national collegiate athletic association athletes from 2009–2010 to 2013–2014: symptom prevalence, symptom resolution time, and return-to-play time. Am J Sports Med. 2016;44(1):226–33. https://doi.org/10.1177/0363546515610537.
21. Vinger PF. A practical guide for sports eye protection. Phys Sportsmed. 2000;28(6):49–69.
22. Kelly SP. Serious eye injury in badminton players. Br J Ophthalmol. 1987;71(10):746–7.
23. Millard L, Breukelman GJ, Mathe N, Shaw I, Shaw BS. A review of the essential visual skills required for soccer: beyond 20–20 optometry. Front Sports Act Living 2022;4 965195. Accessed 30 July 2023. https://www.frontiersin.org/articles/10.3389/fspor.2022.965195

24. Burris K, Liu S, Appelbaum L. Visual-motor expertise in athletes: insights from semiparametric modelling of 2317 athletes tested on the Nike SPARQ Sensory Station. J Sports Sci. 2020;38(3):320–9. https://doi.org/10.1080/02640414.2019.1698090.
25. Knöllner A, Memmert D, von Lehe M, Jungilligens J, Scharfen HE. Specific relations of visual skills and executive functions in elite soccer players. Front Psychol. 2022;13 960092. Accessed 30 July 2023. https://www.frontiersin.org/articles/10.3389/fpsyg.2022.960092
26. Babiloni C, Marzano N, Infarinato F, et al. "Neural efficiency" of experts' brain during judgment of actions: a high-resolution EEG study in elite and amateur karate athletes. Behav Brain Res. 2010;207(2):466–75. https://doi.org/10.1016/j.bbr.2009.10.034.
27. Burris K, Vittetoe K, Ramger B, et al. Sensorimotor abilities predict on-field performance in professional baseball. Sci Rep. 2018;8(1):116. https://doi.org/10.1038/s41598-017-18565-7.
28. Chai WJ, Abd Hamid AI, Abdullah JM. Working memory from the psychological and neurosciences perspectives: a review. Front Psychol. 2018;9 401. Accessed 30 July 2023. https://www.frontiersin.org/articles/10.3389/fpsyg.2018.00401
29. Theofilou G, Ladakis I, Mavroidi C, et al. The effects of a visual stimuli training program on reaction time, cognitive function, and fitness in young soccer players. Sensors. 2022;22(17):6680. https://doi.org/10.3390/s22176680.

Chapter 6
Ophthalmology of Lacrosse

Jay Jaber, William Langston, Julia Doria, and US Lacrosse Official

6.1 Introduction

Lacrosse is one of the oldest and yet fastest growing team sports in the United States [1]. Lacrosse has deep roots in Indigenous tribes' tradition and culture, dating all the way back to the early seventeenth century. While the style of play varied regionally from tribe to tribe, stickball was seen as a ritual as well as a way of training for war. Lacrosse's widespread recognition beyond Indigenous tribes can be attributed to its adoption by European settlers. In 1856, the Montreal Lacrosse Club was founded, marking the beginning of the organized team sport [2].

Through the late 1800s and early 1900s, lacrosse leagues were established in various educational institutions and featured in a few Olympic games, and in 1972 the International Federation of Women's' Lacrosse Association was formed. In 1974, the Men's federation followed suit [2]. From 2012 to 2017, men's college lacrosse has seen a growth rate of 25.8%, while women's has increased by 32.5% [3]. High school participation rates also increased alongside the collegiate level, reflecting the growing popularity of the sport among young athletes. In 2022–2023, the overall high school participant count increased to over 205,000 for both boys and girls nationwide [4].

J. Jaber (✉)
Baylor College of Medicine, Houston, TX, USA
e-mail: Jay.Jaber@bcm.edu

W. Langston
University of Texas San Antonio, Long School of Medicine, San Antonio, TX, USA
e-mail: Langstonw@livemail.UTHSCSA.edu

J. Doria · US Lacrosse Official
USA Lacrosse, Sparks, MD, USA
e-mail: Julia14doria@gmail.com

E. Waisberg et al. (eds.), *Ophthalmology of Sports*,
https://doi.org/10.1007/978-3-031-88645-4_6

6.2 Game Description/Rule Overview

Men's lacrosse is a fast-paced, full-contact team field sport played between two teams of 10. Players use long-handled sticks with mesh pockets, or a "crosse," to catch, carry, and pass the ball, with the objective of shooting it into the opposing team's goal. Defensive players can use a long crosse with an overall length of 52 to 72 inches, whereas offensive players use a short crosse that totals to either 40 or 42 inches in length [5]. Play is initiated through a faceoff between two players of opposing teams at the beginning of each period as well as after every goal. Stick checking and body checking are used to gain possession of the ball and defend the goal. A stick check is performed with the intention of dislodging the ball from an opposing player. Body checking must be done in between the neck and waist from the front or side of an opponent in possession of the ball or within five yards of a loose ball. In this regard, men's lacrosse differs significantly from women's lacrosse, which has a separate set of rules that prohibits body checking and limits overall contact [6].

Women's lacrosse, while it has the same game objectives as men's lacrosse, is played by two teams of 12 and abides by separate regulations that govern other aspects such as shooting, checking, and penalty enforcement. Stick checking, unlike in men's lacrosse, is allowed only on the head of the crosse and gloved hands. It is illegal for women's players to initiate stick-to-player contact and use the shaft of their crosse to hit, push, or displace an opposing player. This type of foul is categorized as a cross check and any cross check that occurs to an opponent's shoulders, head, back, or neck will result in a penalty card [7].

6.3 Protective Equipment

Both men's and women's lacrosse require players to wear protective equipment as regulated by both the NCAA and US Lacrosse. Men's lacrosse requires a helmet with a full-face mask, chin strap, and a mouth guard in addition to shoulder pads, arm pads, and gloves (Fig. 6.1a) [8]. While women are also required to wear a mouth guard, their required equipment differs greatly as in place of a helmet, women are required to wear goggles (Fig. 6.1b). Protective eyewear is required, and women's headgear use is optional. All women's headgear products that include integrated eyewear must also meet the ASTM eyewear standard that women's goggles are required to meet [9].

As previously mentioned, there are major differences in how both men's and women's lacrosse operate. Men's lacrosse is composed of 10 players on the field per team with full contact. During games, every player wears a helmet, mouth gaurd, and various pads to protect them from direct contact with other players, known as "checking. In women's lacrosse, the game is composed of 12 players on the field per team, with only "stick checking." Since 2004, girl and women lacrosse players have been mandated to wear eye protection and mouth guards, and in 2017, an optional helmet was allowed to be worn.

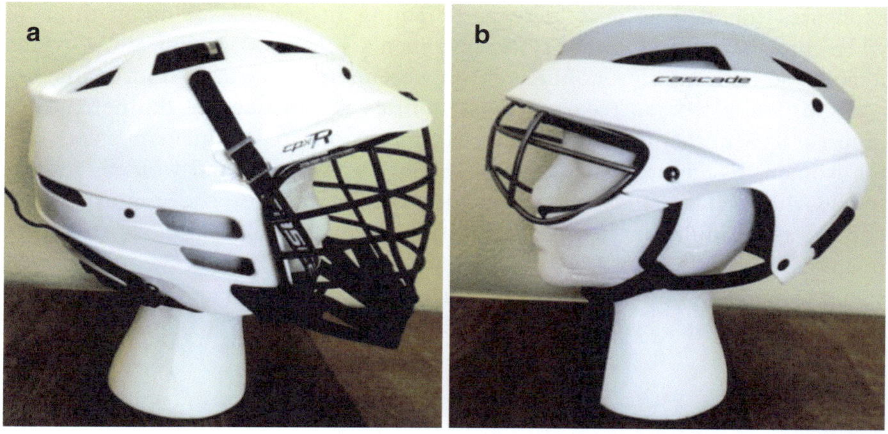

Fig. 6.1 *Part A:* On the left, there is a depiction of the mandated lacrosse helmet for men's lacrosse, with a full-face mask included. *Part B:* The image on the right depicts female protective headgear. Since 2017, female players have had the option to wear protective headgear; however, it is not required [10]. (reprinted from Comstock et al. under Creative Commons Attribution 4.0 International License. https://creativecommons.org/licenses/by/4.0/legalcode)

Table 6.1 The relative increase in youth lacrosse sports from 2006 to 2015 [11]. (Table 6.1 created from data supplied by Kerr et al.)

Youth involvement in lacrosse		
	2006	2015
Girls	81,609	157,061
Boys	139,188	287,519
Overall	220,797	444,580

6.4 The Epidemiology of Ocular Trauma in Lacrosse

As previously stated, the popularity of lacrosse has substantially increased. From 2006 to 2015, participation has doubled, from 220,797 to 444,850. It is important to understand this increase in participation, as more players will inevitably lead to more potential for injuries [11].

Further, above the neck trauma, and specifically ocular trauma, is more prevalent in the female version of the sport. Regardless of the age of play, noted as youth, scholastic or high school, and collegiate, female lacrosse players receive a higher proportion of head and neck injuries compared to their male counterparts [11–14].

6.4.1 Collegiate Lacrosse

On a collegiate level prior to the 2004 season, men's and women's lacrosse players had differences in their total relative head, face, and eye (HFE) injury rates. Men's players were found to have 1.81 HFE injuries out of 1000 athlete exposures (defined as an athlete participating in practice or competition in which they have a risk of injury) to a women's 1.98/1000. In this study, which focused on HFE injuries, collegiate men were more likely to be injured in competition, while women received more injuries in practice. Of the noted HFE injuries, 85% of them were classified as concussions in collegiate men and 41% for women. Eye injuries made up 15% and 19% in men and women, respectively. Although the study did not mention specific diagnoses, eye injuries were defined as an injury including the orbit, eyebrow, eyelid, and other structures related to the eye proper. Importantly, the nature of the cause of the injuries was stated as body-to-body contact in men and stick or ball contact in women. Eye protection in females was mandated in 2004.

6.4.2 Scholastic Lacrosse

Many of the same relationships observed in collegiate lacrosse hold true when analyzing the sport at the high school/collegiate level. In a study encompassing the 2008–2009 to 2015–2016 seasons, the total injuries for high school boys were 20.9 injuries/10,000 athletes. This same statistic was 15.7 injuries/10,000 athletes in high school girls. Injuries in the head and neck region for boys constituted 28.3% of total injuries and high school girls' head and neck injuries made up 29.8%. The most common injury for both parties was concussion. Injuries were generally attributed to contact with another player in boys and contact with a stick or overuse injuries in girls. In this study, it was explicitly mentioned that girl's lacrosse has shown higher rates of eye injuries due to lack of protection in the past [14].

6.4.3 Adolescent and Youth Lacrosse

In a study spanning the 2015–2016 season, youth boy lacrosse players had 12.7 injuries per 1000 athletic exposures in competition and practice. Youth girls had a 8.7/1000 injury rate. The majority of injuries in both males and females occurred during competitive play. A key difference between youth boys' and girls' lacrosse is the mechanism of injury. In competitive play under the age of 13, there is no body checking allowed in boys' play, which is similar to how all levels of girls play the game. Due to this difference, the most common mechanism of injury is due to contact with equipment (contact from sticks or balls). As for body site, the most common injuries in boys were found to be the knee and trunk, with head/face injuries being less common at 8.7%. This contrasted with girls, where head/face injuries were the most prevalent, making up 20.3% of injuries followed by ankle injuries at 15.3%. Of note, 75% of the head/face injuries in girls were due to ball contact.

For both parties, contusions were the most common specific injury. Notably for head/face injuries, concussions were the most common for boys whereas contusions remained the most common for girls (66.7% and 75% of reported head and face injuries, respectively) [11].

6.5 Further Trends

Common considerations for the relative injury rates among sex and skill level are based on multiple factors. First, many of the referenced studies and injuries are reported by athletic trainers in each team's clubhouse. It is likely that many teams across the country do not have full time athletic trainers, and thus there is potential for underreporting of ocular injuries. Second, a lack of penalties called on plays that result in injury have been referenced in multiple studies, calling attention to potential rule changes to enforce penalties which cause injuries. Third, much of the referenced literature is focused on time-stoppage injuries. This trend may indicate further underreporting if a player chooses to wave off an injury in an effort to stay in a game or practice [14].

While many of the cited studies failed to mention the specific eye injuries associated with ocular trauma, lacrosse has been cited as a high-risk sport for ocular trauma among unprotected players. A total of 600,000 sports and recreational related eye injuries occur a year, with 90% being preventable by adequate protection, 42,000 requiring emergency room attention, and 13,500 resulting in permanent vision loss. The most common mechanisms are closed globe, open globe, and radiating injuries. Hyphema is the most common mode of clinical presentation, and objects greater than 5 centimeters in diameter that exert enough force can result in fractures of the thin bones of the orbit floor (lacrosse balls range from 6.27 to 6.47 cm in diameter) [15]. More serious presentations in closed globe injuries include traumatic optic neuropathy, orbital blowout fractures, retinal hemorrhage, vitreous hemorrhage, choroidal rupture, retinal tears, and retinal detachment. Open globe injuries are relatively uncommon [16].

6.6 Considerations for Vision in Lacrosse

6.6.1 Protection

As previously mentioned, one major differentiating factor, the level of contact, helps explain the differences in the use of protective gear for the head and face. While men's lacrosse is a full-contact sport, women's lacrosse consists of limited contact, mainly from lacrosse sticks and balls. Because of the increase in collisions, male lacrosse players are required to wear a full helmet accompanied with a facemask and mouth guard (Fig. 6.2). Female lacrosse players are required to wear protective goggles and a mouth guard but are not required to wear a helmet (Fig. 6.3). Since 2017, an optional helmet now exists for female lacrosse players.

Prior to the 2004–2005 season, female lacrosse players were not required to wear protective eyewear. This changed in 2004, when the United States Lacrosse mandated a new rule, requiring the use of protective eyewear in women's lacrosse. A study conducted in 2012, *Effectiveness of the Women's Lacrosse Protective Eyewear Mandate in the Reduction of Eye Injuries*, compared injury rates from the 2000 to 2003 seasons with injury rates in the 2004–2009 seasons. This study found a significant reduction in injury risk with the introduction of mandated eye protection in women's lacrosse. Without eye protection, the rate of eye injuries was 0.10 out of 1000 athlete exposures. With the introduction of the mandate, the rate of eye injuries dropped to 0.016, or 1.6% of athlete exposures [17]. This significant reduction in eye injuries proved the effectiveness of eye goggles in preventing ocular injury in women's lacrosse.

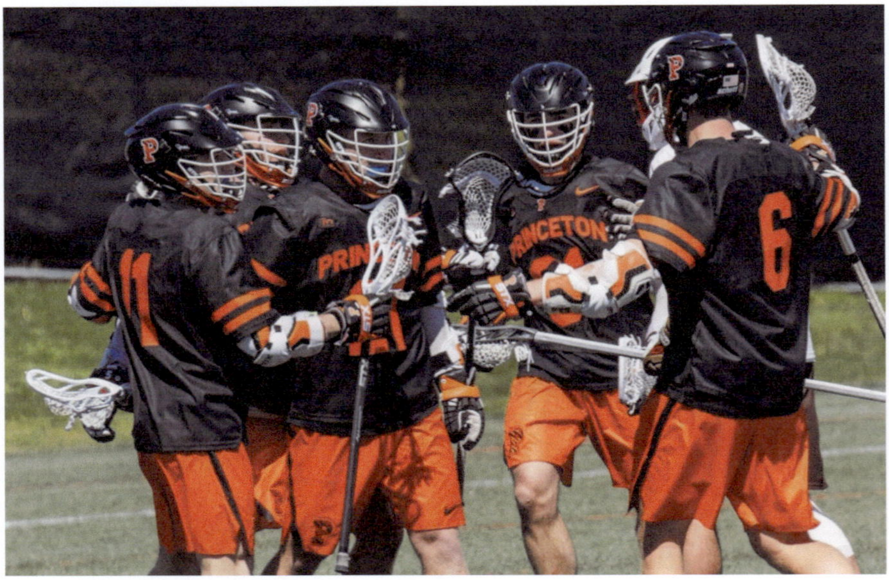

Fig. 6.2 Male collegiate lacrosse players shown wearing lacrosse uniforms. Notice the increased protection afforded to the head by the full helmet and facemask. ("Princeton Tigers Lacrosse players" by Kenneth C. Zirkel is licensed under CC BY-SA 4.0. To view a copy of this license, visit https://creativecommons.org/licenses/by-sa/4.0/?ref=openverse)

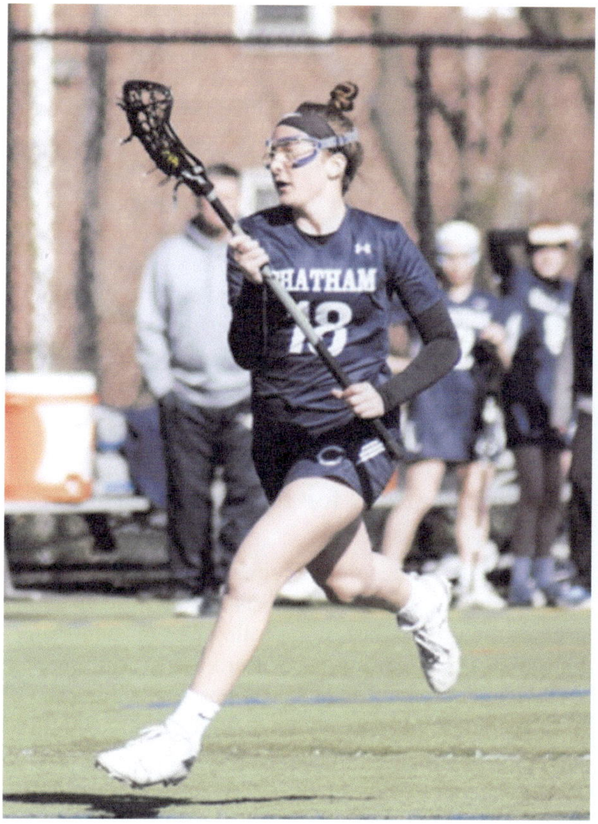

Fig. 6.3 Female scholastic lacrosse player donning the protective eyewear. The use of protective eyewear was not mandated in women's lacrosse until 2004. (Photograph consent provided by Julia Doria. Photo courtesy of image owner and author, Julia Doria)

6.7 Unique Cases

While seemingly rare, ocular injuries can be extremely burdensome to the individual. For example, one adult female's injury sustained during a lacrosse game demonstrates the potential financial burden that can be associated. The immediate medical costs due to the ocular injury amounted to $78,000, with an expectation of additional medical bills in the future [17]. Besides financial repercussions, ocular injuries can significantly alter an individual's quality of life. The importance of vision is difficult to overstate, and long-term vision disturbances are a possible sequela of ocular injury.

While the implementation of mandated eye protection in women's lacrosse has reduced the frequency of eye injuries, it is important to have real-life descriptions of the burden eye injuries have left on patients. Further, while eye protection may be mandated for in-game use, more casual play of all ages may see individuals practicing without their mandated equipment. The following cases display such injuries:

- A 16-year-old girl received an orbital fracture in her right eye after being struck by a ball. Mild enophthalmos was noted. The patient recovered without any sequelae and retained her 20/20 vision.
- A 21-year-old woman sustained hyphema and an iris sphincter tear from a ball striking her right eye. Her vision remained 20/20; however, she has a permanently dilated pupil with photophobia and increased lifetime risk of glaucoma.
- A 19-year-old college woman was struck with a ball and had ecchymosis around the eye. Following a CT scan, inferior and medial wall fractures of the left orbit were noted.
- An 18-year-old woman sustained a right eye contusion after being struck with a lacrosse ball. Periorbital swelling closed her eye, resulting in impaired vision and subconjunctival hemorrhage. There was no orbital bone damage and her vision returned to 20/20 [18].

6.8 Implications for Lacrosse Care

The ability to reduce the incidence of ocular injuries in lacrosse through the use of protective equipment, as well as the significant consequences of ocular injuries, stresses the importance of the following: (1) adherence to rules involving protective equipment, (2) the proper use of protective equipment, (3) the development of better protective equipment, and (4) proper management of ocular injuries.

All lacrosse players, officials, and parents should understand the importance of protective equipment in the prevention of ocular injuries. Rules involving the use of protective equipment should be strictly enforced. Additionally, protective equipment should be worn properly and remain properly worn throughout the entirety of the game and during practices.

More effective protective gear should continue to be engineered and developed over time. An example of this being the introduction of a new lacrosse ball with a 40% reduction in energy transfer in 2017 [11]. Ophthalmologists have a role to play in the research and development of protective gear by assisting in the evaluation of their effectiveness. Ophthalmologists should also be well versed in the treatment of ocular injuries sustained from lacrosse. Treatment should be efficient and conducted in a way that is least burdensome to the patient. Further, ophthalmologists should work in conjunction with primary care physicians, neurologists, and emergency physicians in the management of these injuries, and develop clear plans for their management.

Concussions are the most common type of injury sustained in both men's and women's lacrosse [14]. Concussions are associated with a wide range of complications, including those that affect the eye and vision. One study reported that 82% of patients diagnosed with a concussion had an accompanying ocular motor problem. This included binocular, accommodative, and eye movement complications, with the most common abnormalities being in convergence and accommodation. Out of the patients recommended for visual therapy, only 54% were compliant. Of the compliant patients with convergence issues, 85% were successful and 15% improved. Of the compliant patients with accommodation issues, 33% were successful and 66% improved [19]. These data highlight the importance of increasing the compliance of patients with post-concussive vision disorders, as well as the effectiveness in the treatment of these disorders.

Ophthalmologists should be well versed in the symptoms associated with post-concussive disorders. Early detection and treatment of these disorders can result in full recovery of function and prevent long-term ocular or visual complications. On-site staff (coaches, trainers, administrators) should be aware of the potential visual complications associated with concussions and inform concussed players of treatment options. Primary care and emergency care physicians should be aware of these complications and refer concussed patients to ophthalmologists if there is evidence of ocular or visual damage. Neuro-ophthalmologists have the largest role to play in the treatment of post-concussive visual disorders and should be well versed in appropriate treatment modalities.

References

1. Lacrosse History. USA Lacrosse. Accessed 21 Dec 2023. https://www.usalacrosse.com/lacrosse-history
2. History. World Lacrosse. Accessed 21 Dec 2023. https://worldlacrosse.sport/the-game/origin-history/
3. USLacrosse 2017 Participation survey. https://cdn3.sportngin.com/attachments/document/114e-1909590/Lacrosse_Participation_2017_Survey.pdf
4. High School Athletics Participation Survey 2022–2023. The National Federation of State High School Associations. https://www.nfhs.org/media/7212351/2022-23_participation_survey.pdf
5. 2023 and 2024 Men's Lacrosse Rules Book. The National Collegiate Athletic Association. https://www.ncaapublications.com/productdownloads/LC24-20230124.pdf
6. Women's Field. World Lacrosse. Published November 21, 2023. Accessed 21 Dec 2023. https://worldlacrosse.sport/the-game/disciplines/field-lacrosse/womens-field/
7. 2022 and 2023 Women's Lacrosse Rules Book. The National Collegiate Athletic Association. https://www.usalacrosse.com/sites/default/files/documents/Rules/WLC23.pdf
8. USA Lacrosse Equipment Guide. USA Lacrosse. https://www.usalacrosse.com/sites/default/files/documents/Safety/USAL-equipment-guide-low.pdf
9. Women's Eyewear. USA Lacrosse. Accessed 21 Dec 2023. https://www.usalacrosse.com/womens-eyewear
10. Comstock RD, Arakkal AT, Pierpoint LA, Fields SK. Are high school girls' lacrosse players at increased risk of concussion because they are not allowed to wear the same helmet boys' lacrosse players are required to wear? Inj Epidemiol. 2020;7(1):18. https://doi.org/10.1186/s40621-020-00242-5.
11. Kerr ZY, Lincoln AE, Dodge T, et al. Epidemiology of youth boys' and girls' lacrosse injuries in the 2015 to 2016 seasons. Med Sci Sports Exerc. 2018;50(2):284–91. https://doi.org/10.1249/MSS.0000000000001422.
12. Lincoln AE, Hinton RY, Almquist JL, Lager SL, Dick RW. Head, face, and eye injuries in scholastic and collegiate lacrosse: a 4-year prospective study. Am J Sports Med. 2007;35(2):207–15. https://doi.org/10.1177/0363546506293900.

13. Pierpoint LA, Lincoln AE, Walker N, et al. The first decade of web-based sports injury surveillance: descriptive epidemiology of injuries in us high school boys' lacrosse (2008–2009 through 2013–2014) and national collegiate athletic association men's lacrosse (2004–2005 through 2013–2014). J Athl Train. 2019;54(1):30–41. https://doi.org/10.4085/1062-6050-200-17.
14. Warner K, Savage J, Kuenze CM, Erkenbeck A, Comstock RD, Covassin T. A comparison of high school boys' and girls' lacrosse injuries: academic years 2008–2009 through 2015–2016. J Athl Train. 2018;53(11):1049–55. https://doi.org/10.4085/1062-6050-312-17.
15. Lacrosse Ball Size, Weight, and Diameter. Signature Lacrosse. Published May 19, 2020. Accessed 15 Aug 2023. https://signaturelacrosse.com/blogs/news/lacrosse-ball-size
16. Mishra A, Verma AK. Sports related ocular injuries. Med J Armed Forces India. 2012;68(3):260–6. https://doi.org/10.1016/j.mjafi.2011.12.004.
17. Lincoln AE, Caswell SV, Almquist JL, et al. Effectiveness of the women's lacrosse protective eyewear mandate in the reduction of eye injuries. Am J Sports Med. 2012;40(3):611–4. https://doi.org/10.1177/0363546511428873.
18. Lapidus CS, Nelson LB, Jeffers JB, Kay M, Schwarz DF. Eye injuries in lacrosse: women need their vision less than men? J Trauma. 1992;32(5):555–6.
19. Gallaway M, Scheiman M, Mitchell GL. Vision therapy for post-concussion vision disorders. Optom Vis Sci. 2017;94(1):68–73. https://doi.org/10.1097/OPX.0000000000000935.

Chapter 7
Ophthalmology of Ice Hockey

Ethan Waisberg, Joshua Ong, Mouayad Masalkhi, Ryan J. Daisy, Elizabeth Fortin, and Andrew G. Lee

7.1 Introduction

Hockey is considered the fastest team sport in the world and requires a unique combination of speed, strength, agility, and hand-eye coordination. The sport is continuously growing worldwide, now counting over 1.5 million players, roughly 500,000 of which are located in Canada and 550,000 in the United States [1].

Author, Andrew G. Lee, MD, discloses that he has served or is serving as a consultant for the following companies: AstraZeneca, Alexion, Bristol Mayers Squibb, National Football League, Catalyst, Viridian, Ethyreal, NASA, US Department of Justice, Dompe, and Stoke.

E. Waisberg
Department of Clinical Neurosciences, University of Cambridge, Cambridge, UK

J. Ong
Department of Ophthalmology and Visual Sciences, University of Michigan Kellogg Eye Center, Ann Arbor, MI, USA

M. Masalkhi
University College Dublin School of Medicine, Belfield, Dublin, Ireland

R. J. Daisy
National Hockey League On Ice Official, Buffalo, NY, USA

E. Fortin
Department of Ophthalmology, Neuro-Ophthalmology Service, Massachusetts Eye and Ear, Boston, MA, USA

A. G. Lee (✉)
Department of Ophthalmology, Blanton Eye Institute, Houston Methodist Hospital, Houston, TX, USA
e-mail: aglee@houstonmethodist.org

E. Waisberg et al. (eds.), *Ophthalmology of Sports*,
https://doi.org/10.1007/978-3-031-88645-4_7

While a popular sport, the neuro-ophthalmic principles that impact ice hockey players are not well defined in relation to the sport's biomechanics. These aspects include dynamic visual acuity, saccades, visual field, vestibulo-ocular reflex, and line-of-sight. In this chapter, we review the neuro-ophthalmic principles which underlie the sport of ice hockey and how these fundamentals play a role in the proficiency of hockey players. The key neuro-ophthalmic principles we have identified to be involved in ice hockey are static and dynamic visual acuity, line-of-sight, visual field, color vision, saccades, and smooth pursuit.

7.2 Static Visual Acuity, Dynamic Visual Acuity, and Vestibulo-Ocular Reflex

Hockey players require excellent visual acuity, especially to visualize the puck. In this section, we discuss different types of visual acuity that play a role in sharply visualizing the puck and teammates while on the ice as well as the vestibulo-ocular reflex. The capacity to detect the details of stationary objects whose images are created on the retina when the viewer and the object are motionless is referred to as static visual acuity (SVA) [2].

Several key elements impact SVA. Some are subject- and stimulus-dependent, whereas others are not [2]. Contrast and brightness are some of the most significant among those that are stimulus-dependent. For example, if there is little contrast between the shape and the surrounding, the shape may have to be larger in order to be seen [2]. Additionally, visual acuity improves when increasing the brightness of the object up to a certain level when glare starts to degrade vision [2].

First coined by Ludvigh and Millerin in 1949, dynamic visual acuity (DVA) is a term used to describe the capacity of the eye to distinguish features of an object when either the object, the observer, or both are in motion [2]. DVA is affected by a number of factors, including age, ambient lighting, velocity of the stimulation, exposure duration, and the luminance contrast of the stimulus [2]. It has been shown that increased velocity of the stimulus lowers a subject's DVA. However, the rates at which DVA starts to noticeably decrease are significantly varied according to numerous studies [2]. DVA is essential to various aspects of life activities (such as driving, reading signs while walking, looking at a moving object etc.). Notably, there is a correlation between a low DVA and an increased rate of road accidents [2]. Moreover, DVA is an important predictor of success in sports such as table tennis and baseball [2]. Hockey is considered to be the fastest team sport in the worldwide, making DVA highly important to track the fast-moving puck and surrounding players while being constantly in motion.

The vestibulo-ocular reflex's (VOR) primary purpose is to sustain visual acuity during head movements by maintaining gaze stability [3]. This is achieved by producing slow-phase eye movements that are in phase but in opposite direction to head movement. The "3-neuron arc"—a main sensory afferent neuron with its body in the vestibular nerve's Scarpa's ganglion, a vestibular nucleus neuron in the ponto-medullary area, and an oculomotor neuron in the III, IV, or VI nuclei of the brainstem—provides the basic neuronal circuitry of the VOR [3]. Maintaining an adequate VOR is critical to sustain gaze stability on the puck, sticks, and other players, etc., while skating rapidly. Poltavski and Biberdorf utilized the Nike SPARQ Sensory Training Station to demonstrate that 69% of variance in the goals scored could be predicted by a hockey player's quicker reaction time to visual stimuli, as well as increased visual memory, visual discrimination, and quicker ability to move between focus of near and far objects [4]. These results showed the importance of visuomotor skills and VOR in hockey.

7.3 Visual Performance of Static vs. Dynamic Visual Acuity

Previous research has demonstrated that DVA tends to deteriorate with increasing age. This decline also seems to start earlier and be more noticeable than the loss of SVA's [2]. DVA improves significantly between the ages of 5 and 15 and then begins to decline beyond the age of 20 [2]. In 1966, Burg presented evidence that revealed that DVA was about 60% worse in adults in their 70 s when compared to the average results for a sample of 20-year-old volunteers [5]. One theory suggests that a decline in retinal sensitivity with age could be the root of the problem [2]. According to the findings of other research, a decrease in speed, efficiency, and increase in latency of pursuit and saccadic eye movements may be other contributing factors to DVA degradation in the aging population [6]. In general, increasing brightness levels has a positive effect on DVA, while a decrease in brightness has a more immediate negative effect, similar to what occurs with SVA [2].

There are some considerations highlight the weakness of using SVA alone to assess the visual system [2]. A lot of the visual cues we must react to in reality are in motion. The SVA tests use letters or symbols shown under conditions of utmost contrast (black on white), although such a high degree of contrast is rarely encountered in daily life [2].

A standard ice hockey rink is 200 ft. long by 85 feet wide, while a hockey puck is only 3 inches in diameter. Having adequate static visual acuity is essential to be able to perceive the puck, and to a lesser extent the location of the goaltender, teammates, and the net. However, since professional hockey players skate at speeds up to 48 km/h and the puck remains in near-constant motion the entire game, it is DVA that is required in most situations to allow good tracking of the puck and nearby players.

7.4 Line of Sight and Visual Field

The field of vision is the region of space that can be perceived concurrently while focusing in one direction [7]. The monocular visual field is divided into two sections: the central vision, which includes the center of fixation and the inner

30 degrees of vision, and the peripheral visual field, which includes the outer 100 degrees, middle 60 degrees, upper 60 degrees, and lower 75 degrees [7]. Visual field testing can be done in a variety of ways, including automated static perimetry, Goldmann kinetic perimetry, and confrontation at the patient's bedside [8]. Hockey visors decrease the intensity of a stimulus that can be perceived by over 4 dB of the far temporal visual field (beyond 60 degrees) [9]. If sports goggles were worn instead, this would cause a similar decrease in the far temporal visual field as well as having an additional monocular nasal lens rim scotoma [9].

In hockey, visual field is crucial in order to be aware of other players nearby without looking directly at them. The players must differentiate whether other players nearby are teammates or opponents while skating and concentrating on the puck. If a hockey player had a poor visual field, they would have to constantly move their head around to perform this task and likely lose sight of the puck and their skating direction. A study by Critelli et al. found that the average visual angle threshold of a hockey player is 11.4 degrees [6]. If this threshold angle was increased, a hockey player would have to tilt their head more downward to see the puck, putting them in a more vulnerable position [6].

7.5 Color Vision

During one of Philipp Grubauer's first practice as goalie for the Colorado Avalanche in the National Hockey League (NHL), he stated out loud that he couldn't see "anything out there" [10]. Grubauer had red-green colorblindness, which made it more difficult for him to visualize jersey colors. His teammate, Tyson Jost, also had colorblindness. While things were difficult to visualize, hockey players with color vision deficiencies have successfully performed in the NHL, evidenced by Grubauer and Jost playing in the best hockey league in the world. In an interview, Jost discusses how he is able to practice despite his color deficiency. He stated that he has trainers put him in white practice jerseys so that he can tell what team he is on, and he also relies on contextual clues, by knowing his linemates he relies less on his ability to differentiate between jersey colors. As the NHL often has alternating dark and light jerseys, color vision deficiencies may not impact players as much since they can use contrast to recognize the patterns on their team jersey; however, these rules do not always apply to more junior leagues, and this has impacted Jost earlier in his career to the point where his team had to switch jerseys because he could not recognize his teammates [10]. As mentioned by Jost, accurate color perception is a critical aspect in hockey to be able to rapidly recognize teammates and the opposing team on the ice for quick decision making, particularly when jersey colors are similar.

The ability to discriminate between photons with distinct spectral compositions, independent of intensities, is known as color vision [11]. Color vision depends on comparing signals from photoreceptors with various spectral sensitivity levels [11].

Several hundred colors may be distinguished by humans with normal color vision [11]. To do this, we employ signals from three different types of cone photoreceptors, whose strongest sensitivity ranges from short (S, 430 nm), medium (M, 530 nm), and long (L, 560 nm) wavelengths, but whose tuning is sufficiently broad that each reacts to light throughout most of the visible spectrum—making human vision "trichromatic" [11]. A mammalian photoreceptor's spectrum sensitivity is governed by the opsin it produces, which is covalently coupled to a chromophore in the outer segment [11]. The arrangement of amino acids in the opsin protein determines this compound's spectrum sensitivity, where any alternations in its sequence may impact its function substantially [12].

7.6 Saccades vs. Smooth Pursuit

Usually, a saccadic eye movement to orient to the item being chased comes before a normal smooth pursuit movement [12]. The chase system then aligns the eye's motion with the object's velocity [12]. Saccadic eye movements that minimize retinal error between the current gaze position and the target halt this movement [12]. Compared to saccades, smooth pursuit has a shorter latency (100–125 ms) [12]. Saccades are essential for hockey players to keep track of the puck, their teammates, as well as the goal and goaltender.

7.7 Eye Injury Risk

In Canada, hockey is the sport with the highest incidence of eye injuries [13]. Previous work by the Canadian Ophthalmological Society in the 1970s led to the usage of certified face protectors by hockey players and high stick rules, which significantly reduced eye injuries [13]. There are two types of masks worn in hockey: a full-face mask (covering the face and chin) or half visors which come in two different sizes (one that extends approximately from the above the eyebrow line to the nose bridge and the other to the tip of the nose). Between 1972 and 1999 in Canada, hockey was reported to have caused 1883 eye injuries and 302 blind eyes [14]. However, it is important to note that no ocular injury has ever been reported in hockey players wearing a full-face mask [14]. This data highly supports the exclusive usage of full-face masks in hockey, yet none of the NHL players wears them unless they sustained an injury to the face that requires extra protection. In the National Hockey League (NHL), players suffered 149 eye/orbital injuries over a 10 season period, resulting in a lost financial value greater than $33 million [15]. Visual function with hockey visors remains very similar to that without protective eyewear, with no difference in visual acuity, contrast sensitivity, Ishihara color vision, or foveal threshold; however, there is a decrease in the temporal crescent threshold [9].

7.8 Concussions Impairing Neuro-Ophthalmic Function

High-speed on ice collisions in hockey may result in a player to suffer from subconcussive head impacts (SCHIs). While these head injuries are lesser in severity then full concussive impacts, their increased frequency is concerning, particularly since they were shown to have cumulative effects. Nowak et al. [16] showed that King-Devick Test performance (which tests what?) was impaired after only 10 soccer-ball headings. This study supports that acute neuro-ophthalmic functional impairment can occur following subconcussive head impacts, which frequently occurs in contact sports such as ice hockey [16]. Hockey players also sustain full concussions that can also lead to long-term effects on cognition among others. Although Hockey Canada banned hitting from behind in the 1985–1986 season, and checking to the head in the 2002–2003 season, full concussions are still very prevalent in hockey. The occurrence of just one moderate-to-severe concussion can significantly impact memory and brain function [17].

7.9 Vision Training

Vision training has been previously utilized in field hockey. Schwab et al. [18] found that visual abilities including choice reaction time and peripheral perception can be ameliorated through visual training. However, further research is required to determine if these improvements will lead to any athletic performance increases.

7.10 Conclusion

All things considered, multiple neuro-ophthalmic principles including line-of-sight, dynamic visual acuity, saccades, visual field, and the vestibulo-ocular reflex are involved in the sport of hockey. Further research is required on how these principles can be optimized to further improve on-ice performance.

Disclosures Dr. Andrew G. Lee is a neuro-ophthalmology consultant for the National Football League (NFL).

References

1. Survey of Players. International Ice Hockey Federation. Accessed December 24, 2022. https://www.iihf.com/en/static/5324/survey-of-players
2. Quevedo L, Aznar-Casanova JA, Aparecido da Silva J. Dynamic visual acuity. Trends Psychol. 2018;26(3).
3. Bronstein AM, Patel M, Arshad Q. A brief review of the clinical anatomy of the vestibular-ocular connections – how much do we know? Eye. 2015;29(2):163–70. https://doi.org/10.1038/eye.2014.262.

4. Poltavski D, Biberdorf D. The role of visual perception measures used in sports vision programmes in predicting actual game performance in Division I collegiate hockey players. J Sports Sci. 2015;33(6):597–608. https://doi.org/10.1080/02640414.2014.951952.
5. Burg A. Visual acuity as measured by dynamic and static tests: a comparative evaluation. J Appl Psychol. 1966;50(6):460–6. https://doi.org/10.1037/h0023982.
6. Critelli K, Demiris V, Klatt BN, Crane B, Anson ER. Facemasks block lower visual field in youth ice hockey. Front Sports Act Living. 2021;3:787182. https://doi.org/10.3389/fspor.2021.787182.
7. Mosquera SA, Verma S, McAlinden C. Centration axis in refractive surgery. Eye Vis. 2015;2(1):4. https://doi.org/10.1186/s40662-015-0014-6.
8. Kedar S, Ghate D, Corbett J. Visual fields in neuro-ophthalmology. Indian J Ophthalmol. 2011;59(2):103. https://doi.org/10.4103/0301-4738.77013.
9. Ing E, Ing T, Ing S. The effect of a hockey visor and sports goggles on visual function. Can J Ophthalmol. 2002;37(3):161–7. https://doi.org/10.1016/S0008-4182(02)80058-8.
10. Ingemi M. How Colorblind NHL Players See The Game. FiveThirtyEight. Published March 28, 2022. https://fivethirtyeight.com/features/how-colorblind-nhl-players-see-the-game/. Accessed 30 Dec 2022.
11. Solomon SG, Lennie P. The machinery of colour vision. Nat Rev Neurosci. 2007;8(4):276–86. https://doi.org/10.1038/nrn2094.
12. Mahanama B, Jayawardana Y, Rengarajan S, et al. Eye movement and pupil measures: a review. Front Comput Sci. 2022;3:733531. https://doi.org/10.3389/fcomp.2021.733531.
13. Pashby T. Eye injuries in sports. J Ophthalmic Nurs Technol. 1989;8(3):99–101.
14. Devenyi R, Pashby R, Pashby T. The hockey eye safety program. Ophthalmol Clin N Am. 1999;12(3):359–66. https://doi.org/10.1016/S0896-1549(05)70113-9.
15. Micieli JA, Zurakowski D, Ahmed IIK. Impact of visors on eye and orbital injuries in the National Hockey League. Can J Ophthalmol. 2014;49(3):243–8. https://doi.org/10.1016/j.jcjo.2014.03.008.
16. Nowak MK, Bevilacqua ZW, Ejima K, et al. Neuro-ophthalmologic response to repetitive subconcussive head impacts: a randomized clinical trial. JAMA Ophthalmol. 2020;138(4):350. https://doi.org/10.1001/jamaophthalmol.2019.6128.
17. Lennon MJ, Brooker H, Creese B, et al. Lifetime traumatic brain injury and cognitive domain deficits in late life: The PROTECT-TBI Cohort Study. J Neurotrauma. 2023;40(13–14):1423–35. https://doi.org/10.1089/neu.2022.0360.
18. Schwab S, Memmert D. The impact of a sports vision training program in youth field hockey players. J Sports Sci Med. 2012;11(4):624–31.

Chapter 8
Ophthalmology of Formula 1

Mouayad Masalkhi, Joshua Ong, Ethan Waisberg, Rahul Kumar, Preston Calvert, Peter J. McKnight, David P. Ferguson, and Andrew G. Lee

8.1 Introduction

In less than a second, a Formula 1 automobile can cover over 90 meters, nearly twice the length of a football field [1]. The sport's fast-paced nature demands that drivers execute precise maneuvers, often with timing down to the millisecond, making the accuracy of their vehicle placement on the track crucial. As such, motorsports, particularly Formula 1 racing, have become increasingly popular spectator sports in the United States. Successful drivers must react to and execute complex visuomotor activities at high speeds, requiring exceptional coordination and focus [2].

Author, Andrew G. Lee, MD, discloses that he has served or is serving as a consultant for the following companies: AstraZeneca, Alexion, Bristol Mayers Squibb, National Football League, Catalyst, Viridian, Ethyreal, NASA, US Department of Justice, Dompe, and Stoke.

M. Masalkhi
University College Dublin School of Medicine, Belfield, Dublin, Ireland

J. Ong
Department of Ophthalmology and Visual Sciences, University of Michigan Kellogg Eye Center, Ann Arbor, MI, USA

E. Waisberg
Department of Clinical Neurosciences, University of Cambridge, Cambridge, UK

R. Kumar
Department of Biochemistry and Molecular Biology, University of Miami Miller School of Medicine, Miami, FL, USA

P. Calvert
Department of Neurology, Johns Hopkins School of Medicine, Baltimore, MD, USA

E. Waisberg et al. (eds.), *Ophthalmology of Sports*,
https://doi.org/10.1007/978-3-031-88645-4_8

Additionally, throughout the race, athletes experience significant acceleration forces, particularly during cornering and breaking, where they may face G-forces exceeding four times that of Earth's gravity [3–5]. These G-forces occur when the car changes speed or direction rapidly, as in high-speed cornering or sudden braking. Such forces cause the driver's head, neck, and shoulders to endure increased strain, as the muscles of the neck and shoulders must counteract the forces of the head and helmet [5]—together weighing approximately 6.5 kg [6]. As the G-forces increase, the load on these muscles escalates, which places additional stress on the cervical spine and upper body [7]. Consequently, racing drivers focus on strengthening their neck and shoulder muscles to counteract the physical demands placed on these areas during the race [8, 9]. Extreme decelerations, especially during high-speed cornering or when braking, subject the driver's internal organs, head, and neck to rapid forces that may result in injury [4]. This is particularly true in the event of a crash or sudden deceleration during braking. The rapid change in velocity can cause a range of injuries, including closed head trauma, concussion, and white matter shear injury [3–5, 7, 8]. While aortic dissection could, in theory, occur due to severe deceleration causing blunt trauma [10], modern Formula 1 safety systems have been designed to significantly reduce this risk. Advanced restraint systems, including the 5- and 6-point harnesses, seat designs, and head-and-neck support devices (HANS), are specifically engineered to limit the forces transferred to critical areas of the body, such as the chest and neck, in the event of a crash [11]. These systems ensure that the forces generated by deceleration are distributed more evenly, preventing injuries like aortic dissection. Consequently, while aortic dissection remains a concern in other high-risk activities, it is now considered highly unlike in contemporary F1 racing due to the effectiveness of these safety measures [12].

In addition to physical demands, several key neuro-ophthalmic principles play a vital role in the performance of Formula 1 athletes. These include visual processing speed, hand-eye coordination, depth perception, distance estimation, peripheral awareness, eye tracking (saccades and pursuit), vestibular-ocular reflex (VOR), VOR suppression, gaze stabilization, and accommodation [13–15]. In this review, we explore the core visual and neurophysiological skills required for racing, their impact on performance, and how these factors may inform safety measures and training protocols for drivers.

P. J. McKnight
Hintsa Performance Middle East Consultancy L.L.C., Abu Dhabi, United Arab Emirates

D. P. Ferguson
Department of Kinesiology, Michigan State University, East Lansing, MI, USA

A. G. Lee (✉)
Department of Ophthalmology, Blanton Eye Institute, Houston Methodist Hospital, Houston, TX, USA
e-mail: aglee@houstonmethodist.org

8.2 Core Visual Skills for Racing

8.2.1 Visual Processing Speed and Blinking Speed

Visual processing speed (VPS), or the time required to evaluate and respond to visual stimuli, plays a crucial role in high-speed sports such as racing [16, 17]. VPS encompasses various visual tasks, including identifying targets, distinguishing between, and determining their identity and position [18]. In motorsports, where decisions must be made in fractions of a second, the ability to rapidly process visual information is critical for both performance and safety. Driver reaction time is directly linked to VPS, with faster visual processing enabling quicker decision-making and more precise execution under pressure [18, 19].

Similarly to motorsport competitors, fighter pilots are trained to respond to rapidly changing visual stimuli in the cockpit, and their VPS is crucial for identifying and responding to aerial threats [3, 16, 17, 20]. While these studies do not directly measure Formula 1 drivers, we can speculate that similar principles apply to racing, where drivers must also process rapidly changing visual information. For instance, baseball players rely on VPS to track pitches and respond within milliseconds. Studies have shown that athletes with superior VPS perform better in these dynamic, high-stakes environments [3, 16, 17, 20]. As such, it is reasonable to hypothesize that Formula 1 drivers would also benefit from enhanced VPS, although direct measurements in this population are lacking. Racing drivers are trained to suppress visual behaviors that could disrupt their ability to process visual input continuously [1]. One of the most important strategies is blink suppression, as blinking can temporarily obstruct visual data [21]. By reducing blink frequency, drivers can maintain a continuous visual stream of information, which is crucial when navigating tight corners or traffic on the racetrack.

Alongside blink suppression, drivers employ saccade suppression to maximize the use of their visual field [22]. Saccades are rapid, involuntary eye movements that occur when shifting focus between different points. In racing, drivers need to suppress these saccades and fixate on specific critical points, such as the apex of a turn or brake markers. Suppressing saccades reduces the duration of transient visual input loss, which typically lasts between 20 and 200 milliseconds [23, 24], and ensures that drivers maintain consistent situational awareness on the track.

At speeds such as 210 mph (308 feet per second) in Formula 1 [1], brief lapses in visual input can have significant consequences. For example, during a 200 ms saccadic interruption, a driver can cover 6.2 to 61.6 feet of track, which could be critical in a braking zone. Braking markers are typically placed 300–400 meters before the turn's apex, with 100 meters between each marker pair. The maximum duration of a saccade (200 ms) means that the driver could lose visual input over about 1/5 of the distance between markers—leading to potential uncertainty when deciding when to brake, especially at such high speeds [25].

8.2.2 *Hand-Eye coordination*

Hand-eye coordination (EHC) is a complex motor skill that integrates visual processing with manual control, enabling precise, coordinated actions [26]. In high-performance motorsports, EHC is not merely a prerequisite for skillful driving but a critical factor in maintaining control and safety [27]. The rapid execution of steering, braking, and throttle adjustments requires the precise synchronization of eye movements and manual control, which allows drivers to react instinctively and adapt to the ever-changing environment on the track.

At its core, EHC in racing involves acquiring visual information and translating it into motor actions, with a focus on accuracy and timing. For instance, a driver must continually shift their gaze to points of interest before initiating corresponding hand and body movements to steer and control the vehicle [28]. This sequence is governed by the need to continuously update spatial awareness, requiring the driver's eyes to focus on specific reference points, while the hands move the vehicle in real-time [29]. Saccadic eye movements, which are rapid, involuntary shifts of the eye to a new point of focus [22–25], play a critical role in this process. During a race, drivers must rely on these saccades to transition between multiple track markers—such as braking zones, apexes, and turn exits—aligning visual attention with the hands' movements [26, 27]. The visual system achieves this by focusing the fovea, the region of the retina responsible for high-acuity vision, on a specific point, allowing the driver to assess key track elements with precision [30].

This relationship between visual focus and motor control is evident in the way drivers manage their visual input during high-speed maneuvers. Upon approaching a corner, for example, a driver will shift their gaze from a distant braking marker to the apex of the turn. This gaze shift, or saccade, is followed by the stabilization of visual input at the apex, enabling the driver to smoothly adjust the steering wheel, often accompanied by changes in throttle or brake pressure [21–30]. If done correctly, the driver can ideally guide the car smoothly along the track with minimal deviation. As such, the ability to maintain visual continuity while coordinating upper-body movements and pedal inputs (throttle and brake) is a hallmark of skilled driving and is built through extensive training and repetition [28]. In fact, most Formula 1 drivers start their racing careers by developing basic skills in eye-hand coordination, visual processing, and reactive decision-making [31]. By the time they transition to high-performance vehicles in their teens, they have refined these skills through years of practice, which allows them to maintain control of the car under extreme conditions [29].

From a neurological standpoint, the successful execution of EHC in racing is supported by multiple regions of the brain, including the frontal and parietal cortices, basal ganglia, cerebellum, and brainstem [26]. These areas are involved in visual-spatial processing, eye movement control, and the integration of sensory inputs to guide motor actions. In particular, the basal ganglia and cerebellum coordinate motor execution, while the parietal cortex processes spatial information necessary for directing both eye and hand movements [32]. The integration of VPS with

EHC is particularly important in motorsports [1, 9, 24, 29], without which a driver would be unable to react swiftly enough to changing conditions on the track, leading to suboptimal performance or even accidents.

8.2.3 Dynamic Visual Acuity

Dynamic visual acuity (DVA) refers to the ability to perceive and identify fine details of a moving object despite relative motion between the object and the observer [33]. This skill is essential for motorsports drivers who are in constant motion, and the ability to maintain visual clarity while navigating turns, overtaking other cars, and responding to changing track conditions can be the difference between winning and losing.

DVA can occur under three primary conditions: (1) when the observer's head remains stationary, the object moves, (2) when both the observer and object are in motion relative to one another, or (3) when the object remains stationary but the observer's head or body rotates [34–36]. In motorsports, the third scenario—when both the car and driver are in motion—is the most relevant. During high-speed cornering or acceleration, the driver's eyes must continually adjust to new points of focus, including the apex of turns, brake markers, and nearby competitors, all while the car is undergoing rapid changes in velocity and direction.

The vestibulo-ocular reflex (VOR) plays a crucial role in stabilizing visual input during head movement [37]. This reflex helps the eyes counteract head rotation by generating eye movements in the opposite direction, thereby ensuring that the image remains stable on the retina [38]. While not directly measured in Formula 1 drivers, we can hypothesize that during the intense G-forces experienced in high-speed cornering, as when Formula 1 drivers endure up to 4G [1], the VOR would allow drivers to maintain their focus on critical visual targets even when their heads are moving [37–39]. However, DVA is not solely dependent on the VOR. It is influenced by the gravitational forces acting on the driver's body during acceleration, cornering, and deceleration. When subjected to high G-forces, visual acuity can decrease, resulting in a temporary reduction in the ability to discern fine details [40, 41]. Astronauts, for example, experience diminished DVA during G transitions after returning to Earth, due to the physiological effects of microgravity and re-entry [42]. Similarly, Formula 1 drivers undergo significant G-force transitions during cornering and braking [1, 5, 9], which can affect their ability to maintain sharp visual focus, especially when subjected to abrupt changes in direction and speed.

DVA is neurologically supported by the frontal and parietal cortices for spatial awareness and motor planning and the cerebellum for coordinating motor movements and eye adjustments [14]. DVA integrates reflex systems like the vestibular collic reflex (VCR) and cervicollic reflex (CCR), stabilizing the head and neck during rapid movements [26]. Elite drivers develop DVA through extensive training, which enhances visual-motor coordination, allowing precise, anticipatory control of the vehicle [33].

8.2.4 Stereopsis, Depth Perception, and Distance Estimation

Stereopsis, depth perception, and distance estimation play crucial roles in visual processing for high-speed motorsports. Binocular vision enables drivers to accurately gauge the relative distance and speed of objects, enhancing spatial awareness and improving reaction times [43]. This is particularly important in racing, where drivers must rapidly estimate distances between vehicles and objects in complex, dynamic settings. Studies have shown that stereopsis is especially important in catching performances and interceptive actions typical in sports like tennis, badminton, baseball, and cricket [33]. In team sports with strategic elements, dynamic stereopsis is primarily involved in perceiving depth while following moving subjects or objects [33]. While monocular vision is a disqualifying factor for F1 participation, the evidence supporting the exclusion of monocular drivers in motorsports is not conclusive. A study comparing monocular and binocular truck drivers found that monocular drivers were not significantly worse than binocular drivers in most day-to-day driving functions, despite some reductions in visual capabilities [44]. While this study does not directly measure Formula 1 drivers, it suggests that the impact of monocular vision on driving performance may be complex and context-dependent. Fortunately, research on Monocular Generalized Reduction in Vision (MRV) in competitive driving environments has provided more direct insights. Experiments have shown that drivers under monocular conditions are 2.1 to 6.5 times more likely to collide with target vehicles compared to their baseline (binocular) condition, depending on the driving situation [45]. The study also found an average increase in reaction time from 64 ms to 126 ms under monocular conditions [45]. Interestingly, simulated MRV, which preserved peripheral vision, showed less pronounced effects on reaction times and accident rates compared to complete monocularity [45]. This suggests that preserving peripheral vision may help mitigate some of the adverse effects of reduced visual acuity in racing conditions. These findings underscore the complex relationship between visual conditions and racing performance. While monocular vision may pose significant disadvantages in high-speed motorsports, peripheral vision appears to offer compensatory benefits that can help reduce some of the risks associated with reduced central vision [46]. However, it is important to note that these conclusions are largely based on studies not specific to Formula 1 racing, and further research is needed to confirm these effects in the context of high-speed motorsports.

8.2.5 Peripheral Visual Field

The peripheral visual field is essential for spatial awareness, allowing drivers to detect objects and hazards without shifting their focus [29]. In Formula 1 racing, where drivers navigate at speeds exceeding 200 mph, the ability to maintain a wide visual field is critical for both safety and performance [47]. In humans, the normal binocular field spans about 140°, enabling drivers to anticipate changes in their environment, such as approaching vehicles or obstacles, without directly focusing on them [30]. Studies on peripheral vision in road drivers suggest that visual field deficits can affect safety. For example, a North Carolina study of 52,000 drivers found that those with a visual field of less than 120° were 50% more likely to experience side-impact collisions, despite no difference in overall crash rates [48]. This highlights the importance of peripheral vision in detecting side threats, which could have critical implications for high-speed motorsports. However, Formula 1 drivers face a unique set of challenges. The cockpit design, while optimized for safety, limits peripheral vision due to the fixed seating position and car frame [49]. While peripheral vision deficits in road drivers have been linked to slower reaction times and increased collision risk, the impact of these deficits in motorsports remains underexplored [50]. Glaucoma patients, who suffer from peripheral vision loss, exhibit slower hazard response times, a finding that could be relevant to F1 drivers where rapid reaction to changing conditions is crucial [51]. Adrian's research on Monocular Generalized Reduction in Vision (MRV) provides insights into the effects of vision loss on driving performance, although not specifically in Formula 1 drivers. In his study of 75 drivers, including professionals, those with simulated monocular vision were 2.1 to 6.5 times more likely to collide with other vehicles, with a significant increase in reaction times [45]. While not directly applicable to Formula 1, this suggests that peripheral vision loss, even in less extreme forms than monocularity, could potentially impair a driver's ability to react quickly in a high-speed environment like F1 racing. However, further research specific to Formula 1 drivers would be needed to confirm this hypothesis.

8.2.6 Saccade and Pursuit

Smooth pursuit and saccadic eye movements are critical for tracking moving objects and quickly shifting focus in high-speed environments like Formula 1 racing [52]. Smooth pursuit tracks slow-moving objects steadily, while saccades are rapid eye movements used to shift focus between different points [23]. However, during saccades, visual suppression occurs, meaning no visual information is recorded, resulting in brief blind spots [53]. These movements account for 10–15% of daily visual processing time, which can significantly affect situational awareness during high-speed driving [54]. During saccades, the eye lags behind the moving target for about 120 ms, leading to retinal slip, where the eye's velocity does not match that of the target [29]. To compensate, the eye rapidly accelerates to "catch up," bringing the target into focus on the fovea, the part of the retina responsible for sharp vision [45]. These rapid eye movements allow drivers to focus on essential track features but also create moments of visual disruption, especially in high-speed racing [54]. Once the eye aligns with the target, it enters the steady-state pursuit phase, where the eye matches the target's velocity [55]. This steady tracking is vital for maintaining focus on competitors, braking zones, and other dynamic elements during racing. However, even slight delays in saccadic corrections or pursuit movements can hinder a driver's ability to respond to sudden changes in the environment, like hazards or other cars on the track [29]. In Formula 1, where drivers navigate at speeds over 200 mph, mastering saccades and smooth pursuit is crucial for reaction times and spatial awareness [47]. The ability to suppress unnecessary saccadic movements and optimize pursuit helps drivers maintain continuous visual tracking of track features and competitors, reducing the risk of missed cues or delayed reactions [28].

8.2.7 Enhanced Peripheral Awareness

Peripheral awareness refers to the ability to process environmental information outside the driver's central focus while maintaining attention on the primary path ahead [56]. This skill is essential for Formula 1 drivers, allowing them to sense the flow of the race, track other vehicles, and anticipate changes in track conditions without losing focus on their primary task [57]. In high-speed racing, enhanced peripheral awareness enables drivers to "see everything at once," processing the positions of competitors, potential hazards, and track features in real-time [58]. This ability allows for proactive decision-making—such as blocking overtakes and avoiding collisions—by reacting to competitors approaching from blind spots or adjusting positioning based on peripheral cues [59].

8.2.8 Eye Tracking and Movement Precision

Eye tracking is an essential skill for Formula 1 drivers, allowing them to process rapidly changing visual cues while maintaining control of the car [60]. Unlike everyday driving, where focus is primarily on the road ahead, racing drivers must manage their gaze to track both near and distant objects simultaneously, optimizing their reactions and steering inputs in real-time [61]. A pivotal study by Land and Lee (1994) first demonstrated that non-racing drivers typically focus on the tangent point when navigating curves, which helps predict the direction of the turn and guide steering input [62]. However, Formula 1 drivers utilize multiple fixation strategies, including frequent shifts in gaze between the apex, braking zones, and other cars on the track [57] (Fig. 8.1).

Research by van Leeuwen et al. (2017) using eye-tracking data from a racing simulator revealed that Formula 1 drivers employ a strategy known as "steering with the head," where the head position leads the gaze direction [63]. This strategy contrasts with the tangent-point fixation used by non-racing drivers.

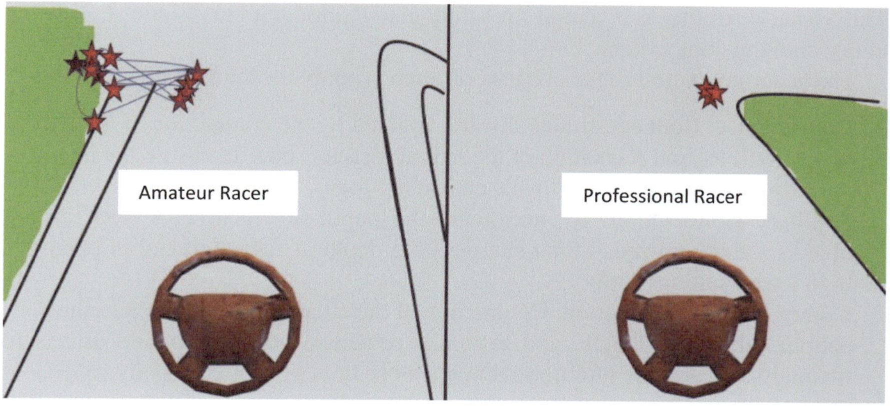

Fig. 8.1 Eye movement patterns for amateur (left) and professional (right) drivers when approaching a turn. In the left panel, amateur drivers exhibit multiple scattered fixations near the road's edge, represented by red stars and connected by blue lines, indicating a shorter, more reactive gaze pattern focused on nearby points. In contrast, the right panel illustrates the professional driver's gaze directed at a single tangent point further along the turn

8.2.9 Focusing and Saccadic Prioritization

In high-speed racing, the ability to rapidly shift focus between near and far objects is critical for spatial awareness and timely responses [64]. Research shows that 80% of sensory input in sports derives from visual information, emphasizing the significance of rapid visual processing in dynamic, high-stakes environments like Formula 1 [65]. This combination of rapid focus shifts, depth perception, and timing coordination distinguishes top drivers, who excel at aligning their responses to the fast-evolving demands of the track.

8.2.10 Accommodation and Convergence

Accommodation refers to the eye's ability to adjust the crystalline lens to focus on objects at varying distances, enabling drivers to quickly shift focus from the circuit ahead to their car's instrument panel or other nearby objects [62]. This accommodation-convergence reflex involves several processes: pupillary constriction, convergence, and ciliary muscle contraction. The reflex pathway includes the optic nerve on the afferent side (similar to the pupillary light reflex) and the oculomotor nerve along with the Edinger-Westphal nucleus on the efferent side [66].

In high-speed racing, accommodation is critical. Drivers must maintain sharp focus on the track while simultaneously monitoring near-field elements, such as speed indicators, in rapidly changing environments and varying light conditions.

This visual flexibility is essential for safely navigating tight curves and responding to fast-moving competitors.

The accommodation reflex consists of three primary mechanisms [66]:

1. Convergence: Both eyes rotate inward, enabled by the contraction of the medial rectus muscles and relaxation of the lateral recti muscles, to ensure the image of a nearby object falls on the fovea, enhancing focus.
2. Pupillary Constriction: By narrowing the pupil, divergent rays from distant objects are minimized, which sharpens the depth of focus, crucial in complex, high-speed settings [66].
3. Ciliary Muscle Contraction: Contraction of the ciliary muscles thickens the lens, shortens the focal length, and increases refractive power, allowing drivers to maintain a clear view of objects that are close or approaching rapidly [66].

8.3 Conclusion

In Formula 1 racing, a driver's success hinges on a complex interplay of neuro-ophthalmic skills, motor coordination, and rapid decision-making under extreme physical demands. Unlike in other high-performance sports, Formula 1 drivers must process visual information with unmatched speed and precision to assess track conditions, anticipate competitor maneuvers, and respond instantly to dynamic changes. Core visual skills—such as dynamic visual acuity, hand-eye coordination, and precise timing integration—enable drivers to maintain situational awareness and perform under intense G-forces and high speeds, where every millisecond is crucial.

The visual reflexes and adaptive mechanisms fundamental to racing, including the vestibulo-ocular reflex and the accommodation-convergence response, play an essential role in stabilizing vision and allowing drivers to quickly shift focus across multiple distances. These processes, supported by pupillary adjustments and ciliary muscle contractions, allow drivers to navigate complex visual fields, from close cockpit displays to distant track markers, without losing visual accuracy or stability.

Advanced gaze strategies, such as anticipating the tangent point and employing head-steering coordination, distinguish elite drivers, enabling them to align visual focus with vehicle dynamics. This anticipatory gaze—an essential skill developed through rigorous training—allows drivers to proactively adjust steering, throttle, and braking inputs to optimize trajectory, anticipate turns, and respond to track conditions and competitors' actions without losing their primary focus on the racing line.

While this review synthesizes findings from various related fields to understand the neuro-ophthalmic demands of Formula 1 racing, it also highlights a significant gap in the literature. Many of the conclusions drawn are based on extrapolations from other high-performance activities or general driving studies. As such, there is a clear need for more direct research on Formula 1 drivers to validate these hypotheses and provide more specific insights into the unique visual and neurological adaptations required for elite motorsport performance. As Formula 1 continues to evolve, understanding these visual and neuromuscular processes will be vital for enhancing both driver performance and safety. Further research in these areas holds the potential to inform training practices and improve racing technologies, ultimately underscoring the importance of neuroscience and biomechanics in optimizing competitive racing.

Disclosures Dr. Andrew G. Lee is a consultant for the National Football League (NFL), NASA, US Department of Justice (DOJ), Horizon, AstraZeneca, and Bristol Myers Squibb.

References

1. Kempema JM. Formula One: a 'crash' course in motorsports medicine. Trauma Surg Acute Care Open. 2024;9(Suppl 2):e001402. https://doi.org/10.1136/tsaco-2024-001402.
2. Carlson LA, Ferguson DP, Kenefick RW. Physiological strain of stock car drivers during competitive racing. J Therm Biol. 2014;44:20–6. https://doi.org/10.1016/j.jtherbio.2014.06.001.
3. Soh MS, Jang JH, Park JS, Shin JH. Effects of high-gravity acceleration forces and anti-gravity maneuver on the cardiac function of fighter pilots. Sci Rep. 2024;14(1):8749. https://doi.org/10.1038/s41598-024-59274-2.
4. Toney-Butler TJ, Varacallo M. Motor vehicle collisions. [Updated 2023 Aug 28]. In: StatPearls [Internet]. Treasure Island: StatPearls Publishing; 2024. Available from: https://www.ncbi.nlm.nih.gov/books/NBK441955/.
5. Weaver CS, Sloan BK, Brizendine EJ, Bock H. An analysis of maximum vehicle G forces and brain injury in motorsports crashes. Med Sci Sports Exerc. 2006;38(2):246–9. https://doi.org/10.1249/01.mss.0000184773.07870.5e.
6. Zoaktafi M, Choobineh A, Rostami M, Kazemi R. The relationship between helmet weight, cognitive performance, and mental workload. Basic Clin Neurosci. 2021;12(6):759–66. https://doi.org/10.32598/bcn.2021.1773.1.
7. Rafique D, Heggli U, Bron D, Colameo D, Schweinhardt P, Swanenburg J. Effects of increasing axial load on cervical motor control. Sci Rep. 2021;11(1):18627. https://doi.org/10.1038/s41598-021-97786-3.
8. McKnight PJ, Bennett LA, Malvern JJ, Ferguson DP. V˙O2peak, body composition, and neck strength of elite motor racing drivers. Med Sci Sports Exerc. 2019;51(12):2563–9. https://doi.org/10.1249/MSS.0000000000001961.
9. Baur H, Müller S, Hirschmüller A, Huber G, Mayer F. Reactivity, stability, and strength performance capacity in motor sports. Br J Sports Med. 2006;40(11):906–10.; discussion 911. https://doi.org/10.1136/bjsm.2006.025783.
10. Fogleman L, Caffery T, Gruner J, Tatum D. Thoracic aortic transection resulting in a type B dissection following blunt trauma. BMJ Case Rep. 2017;2017:bcr2016218766. https://doi.org/10.1136/bcr-2016-218766.
11. Olney DB, Marsden AK. The effect of head restraints and seat belts on the incidence of neck injury in car accidents. Injury. 1986;17(6):365–7. https://doi.org/10.1016/0020-1383(86)90070-7.
12. Hu J, Reed MP, Rupp JD, Fischer K, Lange P, Adler A. Optimizing seat belt and airbag designs for rear seat occupant protection in frontal crashes. Stapp Car Crash J. 2017;61:67–100. https://doi.org/10.4271/2017-22-0004.
13. Schubert MC, Zee DS. Saccade and vestibular ocular motor adaptation. Restor Neurol Neurosci. 2010;28(1):9–18. https://doi.org/10.3233/RNN-2010-0523.

14. Somisetty S, Das JM. Neuroanatomy, vestibulo-ocular reflex. [Updated 2023 Jul 25]. In: StatPearls [Internet]. Treasure Island: StatPearls Publishing; 2024. Available from: https://www.ncbi.nlm.nih.gov/books/NBK545297/.
15. Ventura R, Balcer L, Galetta S. The neuro-ophthalmology of head trauma. Lancet Neurol. 2014;13:1006–16. https://doi.org/10.1016/S1474-4422(14)70111-5.
16. Hülsdünker T, Ostermann M, Mierau A. The speed of neural visual motion perception and processing determines the visuomotor reaction time of young elite table tennis athletes. Front Behav Neurosci. 2019;13:165. https://doi.org/10.3389/fnbeh.2019.00165.
17. Poltavski D, Biberdorf D. The role of visual perception measures used in sports vision programmes in predicting actual game performance in Division I collegiate hockey players. J Sports Sci. 2015;33(6):597–608. https://doi.org/10.1080/02640414.2014.951952.
18. Owsley C. Visual processing speed. Vis Res. 2013;90:52–6. https://doi.org/10.1016/j.visres.2012.11.014.
19. Hülsdünker T, Mierau A. Visual perception and visuomotor reaction speed are independent of the individual alpha frequency. Front Neurosci. 2021;15:620266. https://doi.org/10.3389/fnins.2021.620266.
20. Lounis C, Peysakhovich V, Causse M. Visual scanning strategies in the cockpit are modulated by pilots' expertise: a flight simulator study. PLoS One. 2021;16(2):e0247061. https://doi.org/10.1371/journal.pone.0247061.
21. Berman BD, Horovitz SG, Morel B, Hallett M. Neural correlates of blink suppression and the buildup of a natural bodily urge. NeuroImage. 2012;59(2):1441–50. https://doi.org/10.1016/j.neuroimage.2011.08.050.
22. Guidetti G, Guidetti R, Manfredi M, Manfredi M, Lucchetta A, Livio S. Saccades and driving. Acta Otorhinolaryngol Ital. 2019;39(3):186–96. https://doi.org/10.14639/0392-100X-2176.
23. Bremmer F, Kubischik M, Hoffmann KP, Krekelberg B. Neural dynamics of saccadic suppression. J Neurosci. 2009;29(40):12374–83. https://doi.org/10.1523/JNEUROSCI.2908-09.2009.
24. Crevecoeur F, Kording KP. Saccadic suppression as a perceptual consequence of efficient sensorimotor estimation. Elife. 2017;6:e25073. https://doi.org/10.7554/eLife.25073.
25. Goettker A, Braun DI, Schütz AC, Gegenfurtner KR. Execution of saccadic eye movements affects speed perception. Proc Natl Acad Sci USA. 2018;115(9):2240–5. https://doi.org/10.1073/pnas.1704799115.
26. Rizzo JR, Beheshti M, Naeimi T, Feiz F, Fatterpekar G, Balcer LJ, Galetta SL, Shaikh AG, Rucker JC, Hudson TE. The complexity of eye-hand coordination: a perspective on cortico-cerebellar cooperation. Cerebellum Ataxias. 2020;7(1):14. https://doi.org/10.1186/s40673-020-00123-z.
27. Wilson M, Stephenson S, Chattington M, Marple-Horvat DE. Eye movements coordinated with steering benefit performance even when vision is denied. Exp Brain Res. 2007;176(3):397–412. https://doi.org/10.1007/s00221-006-0623-3.
28. Lappi O, Rinkkala P, Pekkanen J. Systematic observation of an expert driver's gaze strategy-an on-road case study. Front Psychol. 2017;8:620. https://doi.org/10.3389/fpsyg.2017.00620.
29. Wolfe B, Sawyer BD, Rosenholtz R. Toward a theory of visual information acquisition in driving. Hum Factors. 2022;64(4):694–713. https://doi.org/10.1177/0018720820939693.
30. Provis JM, Dubis AM, Maddess T, Carroll J. Adaptation of the central retina for high acuity vision: cones, the fovea and the avascular zone. Prog Retin Eye Res. 2013;35:63–81. https://doi.org/10.1016/j.preteyeres.2013.01.005.
31. Gordon BR. Behind the visor: a qualitative exploration of the psychological skills of Formula One race car drivers. Master's thesis, Temple University. Temple University Graduate Board. 2015. https://digital.library.temple.edu/
32. Errante A, Fogassi L. Activation of cerebellum and basal ganglia during the observation and execution of manipulative actions. Sci Rep. 2020;10(1):12008. https://doi.org/10.1038/s41598-020-68928-w.
33. Palidis DJ, Wyder-Hodge PA, Fooken J, Spering M. Distinct eye movement patterns enhance dynamic visual acuity. PLoS One. 2017;12(2):e0172061. https://doi.org/10.1371/journal.pone.0172061.

34. Wang X, Yan M, Li J, Wang Y. The short- and long-term perceptual learning of clinical dynamic visual acuity test. Invest Ophthalmol Vis Sci. 2024;65(12):43. https://doi.org/10.1167/iovs.65.12.43.
35. Erdinest N, London N. Dynamic visual acuity and methods of measurement. J Optom. 2022;15(3):247–8. https://doi.org/10.1016/j.optom.2021.06.003.
36. Peters BT, Bloomberg JJ. Dynamic visual acuity using "far" and "near" targets. Acta Otolaryngol. 2005;125(4):353–7. https://doi.org/10.1080/00016480410024631.
37. Fetter M. Vestibulo-ocular reflex. Dev Ophthalmol. 2007;40:35–51. https://doi.org/10.1159/000100348.
38. Simakurthy S, Tripathy K. Oculovestibular Reflex. [Updated 2022 Nov 7]. In: StatPearls [Internet]. Treasure Island: StatPearls Publishing; 2024. Available from: https://www.ncbi.nlm.nih.gov/books/NBK542281/.
39. Jones SM, Jones TA, Mills KN, Gaines GC. Anatomical and physiological considerations in vestibular dysfunction and compensation. Semin Hear. 2009;30(4):231–41. https://doi.org/10.1055/s-0029-1241124.
40. Muzdalo NV. The importance of measuring dynamic visual acuity. Coll Antropol. 2013;37(Suppl 1):275–85.
41. Horng CT, Hsieh YS, Tsai ML, Chang WK, Yang TH, Yauan CH, Wang CH, Kuo WH, Wu YC. Effects of horizontal acceleration on human visual acuity and stereopsis. Int J Environ Res Public Health. 2015;12(1):910–26. https://doi.org/10.3390/ijerph120100910.
42. Mulavara AP, Peters BT, Miller CA, Kofman IS, Reschke MF, Taylor LC, Lawrence EL, Wood SJ, Laurie SS, Lee SMC, Buxton RE, May-Phillips TR, Stenger MB, Ploutz-Snyder LL, Ryder JW, Feiveson AH, Bloomberg JJ. Physiological and functional alterations after spaceflight and bed rest. Med Sci Sports Exerc. 2018;50(9):1961–80. https://doi.org/10.1249/MSS.0000000000001615.
43. Laby DM, Kirschen DG, Pantall P. The visual function of Olympic-level athletes – an initial report. Eye Contact Lens. 2011;37(3):116–22. (44)
44. McKnight AJ, Shinar D, Hilburn B. The visual and driving performance of monocular and binocular heavy-duty truck drivers. Accid Anal Prev. 1991;23(4):225–37.
45. Adrian J, Le Brun J, Miller NR, Sahel J-A, Saillant G, Bodaghi B. Implications of monocular vision for racing drivers. PLoS One. 2019;14(12):e0226308.
46. Bowers AR, Mandel AJ, Goldstein RB, Peli E. Driving with hemianopia, I: detection performance in a driving simulator. Invest Ophthalmol Vis Sci. 2009;50(11):5137–47.
47. International Sports Vision Association. Motorsports – ISVA. [Internet]. 2024 [cited 2024 Nov 13]. Available from: https://www.sportsvision.pro/athletes/dynamic-visual-skills-for-sports/motorsports/
48. McGwin G Jr, Xie A, Mays A, Joiner W, DeCarlo DK, Hall TA, Owsley C. Visual field defects and the risk of motor vehicle collisions among patients with glaucoma. Invest Ophthalmol Vis Sci. 2005;46(12):4437–41.
49. Watkins S, Vino G. The effect of vehicle aerodynamics on the driver's field of view. SAE Technical Paper. 2008;2008-01-0806.
50. Wood JM, Black AA, Mallon K, Thomas R, Owsley C. Glaucoma and driving: on-road driving characteristics. PLoS One. 2016;11(7):e0158318.
51. Glen FC, Smith ND, Crabb DP. Saccadic eye movements and face recognition performance in patients with central glaucomatous visual field defects. Vis Res. 2013;82:42–51.
52. Spering M, Montagnini A. Do we track what we see? Common versus independent processing for motion perception and smooth pursuit eye movements: a review. Vis Res. 2011;51(8):836–52.
53. Lappi O. Future path and tangent point models in the visual control of locomotion in curve driving. J Vis. 2014;14(12):21.
54. Land MF. Eye movements and the control of actions in everyday life. Prog Retin Eye Res. 2006;25(3):296–324.

55. Lisberger SG. Visual guidance of smooth-pursuit eye movements: sensation, action, and what happens in between. Neuron. 2010;66(4):477–91.
56. Land MF, Lee DN. Where we look when we steer. Nature. 1994;369(6483):742–4.
57. Leeuwen PM, de Groot S, Happee R, de Winter JC. Differences between racing and non-racing drivers: a simulator study using eye-tracking. PLoS One. 2017;12(11):e0186871.
58. Wilkie RM, Wann JP. Eye-movements aid the control of locomotion. J Vis. 2003;3(11):677–84.
59. Kandil FI, Rotter A, Lappe M. Driving is smoother and more stable when using the tangent point. J Vis. 2009;9(1):11.1–11.
60. Land MF, Tatler BW. Looking and acting: vision and eye movements in natural behaviour. Oxford University Press; 2009.
61. Salvucci DD, Gray R. A two-point visual control model of steering. Perception. 2004;33(10):1233–48.
62. Charman WN. The eye in focus: accommodation and presbyopia. Clin Exp Optom. 2008;91(3):207–25.
63. van Leeuwen PM, de Groot S, Happee R, de Winter JC. Effects of concurrent continuous visual feedback on learning the lane keeping task. Hum Factors. 2017;59(7):1173–87.
64. Hülsdünker T, Strüder HK, Mierau A. Neural correlates of expert visuomotor performance in badminton players. Med Sci Sports Exerc. 2016;48(11):2125–34.
65. Williams AM, Davids K, Williams JG. Visual perception and action in sport. London: E & FN Spon; 1999.
66. Somisetty S, Das JM. Neuroanatomy, accommodation reflex. In: StatPearls [Internet]. Treasure Island: StatPearls Publishing; 2023.

Chapter 9
Ophthalmology in Football and National Football League (NFL) Officiating

Ethan Waisberg, Joshua Ong, Mouayad Masalkhi, Ashtyn Zapletal, Nicole Carrabba, Nasif Zaman, Prithul Sarker, Alireza Tavakkoli, and Andrew G. Lee

9.1 Introduction

Officials from the early days of professional football would be unrecognizable to fans of today, from wearing black bow ties and dress shirts on-field to using horns to call penalties rather than flags. The level of professionalism exhibited by these early officials was also nowhere near the level it is at today, where officials were

---

Author, Andrew G. Lee, MD, discloses that he has served or is serving as a consultant for the following companies: AstraZeneca, Alexion, Bristol Mayers Squibb, National Football League, Catalyst, Viridian, Ethyreal, NASA, US Department of Justice, Dompe, and Stoke.

E. Waisberg
Department of Clinical Neurosciences, University of Cambridge, Cambridge, UK

J. Ong
Department of Ophthalmology and Visual Sciences, University of Michigan Kellogg Eye Center, Ann Arbor, MI, USA

M. Masalkhi
University College Dublin School of Medicine, Belfield, Dublin, Ireland

A. Zapletal
Texas A&M College of Medicine, Bryan, TX, USA

N. Carrabba
McGovern Medical School at UTHealth, Houston, TX, USA

N. Zaman · P. Sarker · A. Tavakkoli
Human-Machine Perception Laboratory, Department of Computer Science and Engineering, University of Nevada, Reno, Reno, NV, USA

A. G. Lee (✉)
Department of Ophthalmology, Blanton Eye Institute, Houston Methodist Hospital, Houston, TX, USA
e-mail: aglee@houstonmethodist.org

E. Waisberg et al. (eds.), *Ophthalmology of Sports*,
https://doi.org/10.1007/978-3-031-88645-4_9

previously undertrained, inadequately supervised and ill-equipped, helping to contribute to low-scoring games in the early days of the National Football League (NFL) [1]. In 1938, Hugh Ray worked with the NFL to develop a "play situation book" which prepared football officials for any possible scenario that can occur and continues to be used today [1]. With clearly defined rules, football became safer, faster, and more entertaining, leading to a rapid increase in its popularity. As the NFL grew, the officiating crews grew with it, with officials now having a seven-person crew, which is now known for its excellence.

In 2019, a critical error was made in the NFL Conference Championship game between the Los Angeles Rams and New Orleans Saints. Drew Brees, quarterback of the New Orleans Saints, threw the ball towards his wide receiver Tommylee Lewis on the right sideline. Nickell Robey-Coleman of the Rams ran and made high impact into Lewis well before the ball arrived, but no penalty call was made on the field. The New Orleans Saints subsequently were forced to attempt a field goal rather than a touchdown and the Saints were eliminated from the playoffs [2].

Following this officiating error, the NFL reviewed the missed call and fined the Rams player $26,739 for an illegal helmet-to-helmet hit from this play [3]. This play in part also resulted in changes in the instant-replay rules, allowing coaches to challenge pass interference calls or non-calls. This example illustrates the importance of high-quality officiating in the NFL and how sufficient visual information is required for an officiator to make decisions. There are a multitude of aspects that contribute towards a proficient officiator, including the field of neuro-ophthalmology.

Neuro-ophthalmology is a medical subspecialty that focuses on vision that relates to the brain and is a highly applicable field in American football officiating. Fundamental considerations in neuro-ophthalmology including static and dynamic visual acuity, line-of-sight and visual field play a critical role in proficient analysis on the field. In this chapter, we review the current knowledge of ophthalmology in football. We then describe neuro-ophthalmic principles which underlie American NFL football officiating. We also provide an overview of ongoing research that employs these fundamentals in neuro-ophthalmology to optimize NFL officiating.

9.2 Ophthalmology of Football

There is growing concern over the safety and long-term health effects of American football players. Injuries in American football are highly prevalent, and the NFL and its Player Safety Advisory Panel continuously introduce new innovations and technologies to better protect players and advance the game [4]. Neuro-ophthalmic injuries can include concussions, Chronic traumatic encephalopathy (CTE), and eye injuries. Traumatic ocular events and their sequelae can subject patients to potential long-term physical, psychosocial, and economic consequences [5]. Haring et al. [6]

found that 2.9% of all sports-related ocular injuries examined from the Nationwide Emergency Department Sample (NEDS) database from January 1, 2010, and December 31, 2013 were due to football. Patel [7] and colleagues found that out of 4671 sports-related ocular injuries from 2010 to 2019 in the National Electronic Injury Surveillance System All Injury Program (NEISS-AIP) database, football was the third most frequent sport ($n = 576$, 12.3%). Ocular trauma related to football had a significantly greater frequency of corneal or scleral abrasions compared to other sports. Among the 576 football-related ocular injuries, corneal/scleral abrasions made up 41.7%, contusion 11.5%, subconjunctival hemorrhage/hematoma 5.7%, and all others at 41.10% [7].

To prevent such eye injuries from occurring in football, the American Academy of Ophthalmology recommends the use of protective eyewear for all athlete participants in American football. Currently, visor use is optional among player safety recommendations in the NFL [4]. While some players may opt to avoid visor use due to concerns on view obstruction, a previous study found that visor use did not have a significant effect on target detection and reaction time [8]. Dhoot and colleagues [4] found a total of 16 eye injuries sustained from the 2015–2019 to 2019–2019 NFL seasons (including preseason, regular season, and playoffs). These included eye gouges ($n = 6$), orbital fractures ($n = 2$), eye lid lacerations ($n = 1$), and corneal abrasions ($n = 1$). Twelve injuries occurred in players who did not wear visors, and four injuries occurred in players who wore visors. It should be noted that no cause or specific diagnosis was established in the visor-wearing players. This study also found that visor use continued to increase in each year of analysis, which is promising. Though relatively uncommon, these types of eye injuries can have permanent and career-ending consequences. Visors are a safe and effective way to prevent such eye injuries in the NFL.

Over the past few decades, football-related concussions have generated greater public awareness and increased concerns about player safety. The growing body of medical literature suggests that even a single concussion can cause persistent sleep problems, headaches, memory disorders, and reduced attention [9]. Importantly, it is often difficult to assess and characterize concussions accurately and objectively. Consequently, concussions are often underreported and therefore undertreated. Between the years of 2015 and 2019 using the electronic health record (EHR) data based on medical staff reporting, a retrospective, observational study found a total of 1302 concussions, with 80% of them occurring during games. There were 790 regular season game concussions across 114,428 player-games during the five-year study period. The authors found that an average of 243 NFL players suffered concussions per season of playing. This equated to a 7% one-season risk of sustaining one or more concussions [10].

During this period, numerous player safety initiatives to improve identification and reduction of concussions were launched in the NFL. In 2015, a centralized clinical EHR was introduced with reporting audits that scanned and reviewed the data within the system to ensure quality reporting. Efforts to better detect concussions led to the development of AT Spotter [11, 12]. Beginning in the 2018 season, detailed review of every injury along with concussion-focused discussions occurred with every team. In addition, changes in the game rules have been implemented in attempt to reduce high-risk play types. These included restrictions on lowering the head to initiate contact, prohibition of blindside blocks, changes in kickoffs to prevent running starts and wedge blocks [10].

The National Operating Committee on Standard for Athletic Equipment (NOCSAE) sets the standards and criteria for helmet evaluation, and the NFL requires its players to use helmets that meet these NOCSAE standards. Helmets are mandatory in football, and extensive laboratory testing has been conducted to evaluate the quality of different helmet models. This led to the transition to better performing helmet models for nearly all NFL players [10]. One study found that players during the 2018 and 2019 seasons had significantly lower odds of sustaining a concussion when compared to the 2015 season ($p < 0.05$) [13]. The NFL also hosts the NFL Helmet Challenge and funds ongoing research to develop position-specific helmets for future helmet innovation and improvement.

9.3 Neuro-Ophthalmology of NFL Officiating

American football at all levels relies heavily on high quality officiating, and competent, consistent, reliable, and professional game officials are an integral part of the sport at all levels. NFL football involves a seven-person team of officiators. This team consists of a referee, umpire, head linesman, line judge, field judge, side judge, and back judge. Their assigned roles are described in Table 9.1.

Table 9.1 Members of the NFL officiating team and their assigned roles [14]

NFL officiating team member	Assigned role
Referee	Has final say over other officials. Stands behind offence and watches quarterback. Prioritizes making calls on forward passes or roughing the passer. Makes official signals and announcements to crowd and teams. Reviews challenged plays in TV booth
Umpire	Ensures no equipment violations. Responsible for calling line play penalties such as illegal blocks and holding. Also counts offensive players
Head Linesman	Stands in visitor's end
	Responsible for calling all alignment, false start, offsides, pre-snap and neutral-zone penalties
Line Judge	Stands in home team's end. Same role as head linesman. Also manually keeps game time.
Field Judge	Stands on home sideline. Counts defensive players, makes complete/incomplete rulings, and can call out-of-bounds
Side Judge	Stands in visitor's end. Same role as Field judge
Back Judge	Makes rulings on field goal attempts. Times breaks, inter-intermission and halftime periods and notifies teams when to resume playing

Currently 121 officials work in the NFL [15]. These game officials have a cognitively demanding role, being responsible for enforcing in real time every rule from a 245-page Official NFL Playing Rules rulebook. The regulations and rules of the game are continually reviewed and modified as necessary from year to year [16]. NFL game officials also have over 35 hand signals which are used for clear communication. Similar to NFL players, the accuracy of an official's call can be a deciding factor on whether they will advance to work in post-season games. The performance of each game official is also thoroughly reviewed on a weekly basis by the NFL's Officiating Department by supervisors with decades of officiating experience. Officials are typically correct on 98.9% of calls. It is important to note that this figure does not include non-calls. However, even on challenged calls elevated to instant-replay for review, only 40% of these calls have been overturned since 1999 [15].

9.4 Unobstructed Line of Sight and Adequate Visual Field

Football is an extremely fast-paced sport, and maintaining a clear and unobstructed line of sight during the play is particularly challenging when there are 22 players on the field in constant motion. A typical NFL game now averages about 153 plays [15]. The sport continues to become faster-paced, with a 150% increase in no-huddle plays from 2008 to 2013 [15]. The increased speed and quantity of plays increases the possibility for officiating errors to occur. Some officiating calls such as pass interference can be difficult to make and require the timing of contact with players to be constantly observed by officiators.

The area of space where things may be seen simultaneously while looking steadily in one direction is known as the field of vision. The monocular visual field comprises two parts: the central vision, which encompasses the inner 30 degrees of vision and the center of fixation, and the peripheral visual field, which encompasses 100 degrees laterally, 60 degrees medially, 60 degrees vertically, and 75 degrees downwards [17]. There are several methods for performing visual field testing, including confrontation at patient's bedside, Goldmann kinetic perimetry, and automated static perimetry [18].

Line of sight (LOS) is a line from the fixation point that passes through the pupil center (PC) and into the foveola. When compared to the visual axis, the LOS is linked with a significantly longer optical path difference (OPD) [19]. Two light sources, one focused on the retina and the other out of focus, concurrently fixed at varying distances from the eye can be used to calculate LOS [19]. The ray from the out-of-focus source will produce a fuzzy circle, while the beam via PC (the focused source) will form the blur circle's center if the principal rays from both sources overlap and they fall on the LOS [19].

9.5 Static vs. Dynamic Visual Acuity

NFL officials may be required to move during an active play to preserve unobstructed LOS and to watch a developing play with sufficient visual field. The capacity to discern the specifics of static objects whose picture is created on the retina when the assessed topic is also stationary is referred to as static visual acuity (SVA) [20]. The refractive error is one of the main elements that may affect SVA. In most situations, this can be corrected with the right optical prescription. The age of the individual is a crucial component as well because it is known to cause variations (anatomical and physiological) that have a negative impact on visual perception [20].

When an object, the observer, or both are moving, the capacity to visually interpret fine spatial features of the object is known as dynamic visual acuity (DVA) [21]. DVA is described as the capacity to distinguish between an object's features when there is relative motion between the object and the observer [20]. Previous studies have illustrated that DVA is one of the abilities that declines with aging. This decline starts sooner and is more pronounced than SVA [20]. Between the ages of 5 and 15 years, DVA increases significantly, and beyond the age of 20, it starts to decrease [20]. In 1966, Burg demonstrated that, as compared to the typical outcomes for a population of 20-year-old participants, DVA was almost 60% worse in people in their 70s [20]. One theory proposes reduction or loss or retinal sensitivity could be the cause [20]. Other studies suggest decline in speed, efficiency, and latency of pursuit and saccadic eye movement as an underlying cause of DVA deterioration in the elderly population [20]. DVA improves by raising the brightness, but it is more instantly impacted when it lowers, much like what happens with SVA [20]. Thus, as opposed to NFL players who are typically younger, NFL game officials are significantly older individuals with diminished DVA.

9.6 Saccades vs. Smooth Pursuit

NFL officials need to have a deep-understanding of the game to anticipate the actions of the players to better follow the game. Saccadic movements are brief and quick eye movements that enable the observer to perceive an item at a specific area in the visual field and focus it on the fovea, allowing for a greater potential for discrimination [22]. The trajectory or orientation of a series of saccades is a helpful descriptive metric—normally expressed as a relative or absolute value [22]. Calculating relative saccade direction involves comparing the absolute saccade directions of two successive saccades. The absolute saccade direction is binned into pre-specified angular segments to provide discretized saccade directions [22].

Previous research has discovered that complex neural signals in the Superior Colliculus (SC) and Frontal Eye Field (FEF) are necessary for saccade preparation, with the former found to be connected with the pupil control circuit [22]. Game officials, through years of experience and training, learn to optimize their saccadic prioritization during specific plays.

Typically, a typical smooth pursuit movement is preceded by a saccadic eye movement to orient to the object being pursued [22]. The pursuit mechanism then matches the eye's velocity to that of the object [22]. This movement is interrupted by saccadic eye movements that reduce retinal error in between the present gaze location and the target [22]. Smooth pursuit has a shorter delay (100–125 ms) compared to saccades (200–250 ms) [22].

9.6.1 Vergence Movements

As referees need to look into different planes of 3D space, vergence movements play a key role in maintaining adequate vision by allowing the visual target to be focused on the foveae. To focus on a near target, the eyes converge (rotate nasally), while the eyes diverge (rotate laterally) to focus on a distant target. The two most important visual stimuli to trigger vergence movements are retinal disparity and image blur [23]. As vergence movements are relatively slow (1 s or longer), the importance or referees looking at the right part of the field prior to making an important calls is key.

9.6.2 Stereopsis and Monocular Depth Cues

Accurate perception of depth is crucial for an NFL referee when determining player errors in placement or the location of the football. Stereopsis refers to the perception of depth obtained through binocular vision. As each eye is in a slightly different position, this results in a binocular disparity, with this disparity being processed in the visual cortex to produce depth perception. Fine stereopsis is used to determine depth perception in the central area of vision. High levels of static visual acuity is required in both eyes to have high levels of fine stereopsis. Monocular visual cues may also be used by referees to enhance depth perception, such as looking at the size of an object or by motion parallax.

9.7 Fewer Officiating Practice Opportunities

An additional challenge for NFL officiators is that an NFL plays far few games than most major sports, with only 272 total regular season games (17 per team). Sports such as baseball (MLB) have 2430 total regular season games (162 games per team), and basketball (NBA) has a season comprised of 1230 regular season games (82 per team). Thus, individual NFL games have higher stakes and game officials have less real world opportunities to experience NFL gameplay. This decreased opportunity for NFL officiators to acquire experience means that training is essential prior to official game day assignment. Woods et al. [24] showed that as experience with football increases, the accuracy of officiating calls improved significantly, resulting in fewer interference calls, and directional bias of these calls decreased.

A unique example of this in the NFL occurred during the labor dispute in the 2012 season, when NFL officiators decided to lockout. Less-experienced replacement officials then officiated NFL games and became heavily criticized for a multitude of factors including inaccurate clock management, inconsistent penalty calls, and yardage penalization errors [24].

9.8 Fieldwork

To compensate for fewer officiating practice opportunities, emphasis has been placed on two integral practices: video review and training camps. Every week, NFL game officials are expected to review several hours of game footage, looking for areas of improvement. However, video review only provides authenticity to a certain extent and therefore lends itself to potential research in ways to more accurately replicate game play. Additionally, official's training camps attempt to bridge this gap by providing on-field experience, typically during high school football games. Members of our team have been present during this on-field implementation of the above neuro-ophthalmology principles. This real-time repetition provides more immersive exercises and helps to create muscle memory when applying neuro-ophthalmology principles to various football plays. Both aspects of official training were presented during a platform presentation at the 2022 American Academy of Ophthalmology meeting in Chicago, Illinois [25].

9.9 Current Research and Future Direction

The neuro-ophthalmic principles herein were presented by members of our team to 17 head NFL referees, along with other officiating staff. The neuro-ophthalmology curriculum development and implementation were presented previously at the American Academy of Ophthalmology (AAO) annual meeting in 2022. The goal of this curriculum was to increase the understanding of neuro-ophthalmic principles in NFL officiators and improve the accuracy of their calls.

We surveyed the officiating staff's prior knowledge of neuro-ophthalmic terms prior to our presentation. Prior to the presentation, only one referee reported an understanding of these terms. Following the presentation, the knowledge of the group of officials increased significantly [25]. We then examined the likelihood of these senior NFL officials to use these newly learned neuro-ophthalmic terms in the training of future NFL officials. Following the presentation, the referees were much more likely to use these terms [25]. To determine the relevance of these neuro-ophthalmic terms, the NFL officials were then asked to rate the relevance of the presentation. Overall, presentation was rated to be highly relevant by all NFL officials with the lowest score of relevance being 6 out of 10 [25]. About 67% of the official reported having a maximum interest (10 out of 10) in attending future neuro-ophthalmic talks. Based on this feedback, we plan on having further talks on neuro-ophthalmic principles for NFL officials.

Our group is also currently developing a NASA-funded head-mounted visual assessment system to help detect subtle visual changes that occur during spaceflight [26, 27]. In relation to the neuro-ophthalmic fundamentals, we have reported the technical development and pilot study results of head-mounted dynamic visual acuity assessment which have strong implications for NFL officiating assessments [28]. Future applications of this technology terrestrially are to screen populations in developing countries for preventable causes of blindness [29, 30]. Current research is being conducted to validate the head-mounted contrast sensitivity assessments and enhance dynamic visual acuity with augmented reality, both of which have strong applications to NFL officiating. Additionally, our group is also actively developing a virtual reality simulation tool for NFL officiators to more accurately simulate gameplay and provide additional insight between the spectrum of gameplay analysis and on-field experience (Fig. 9.1).

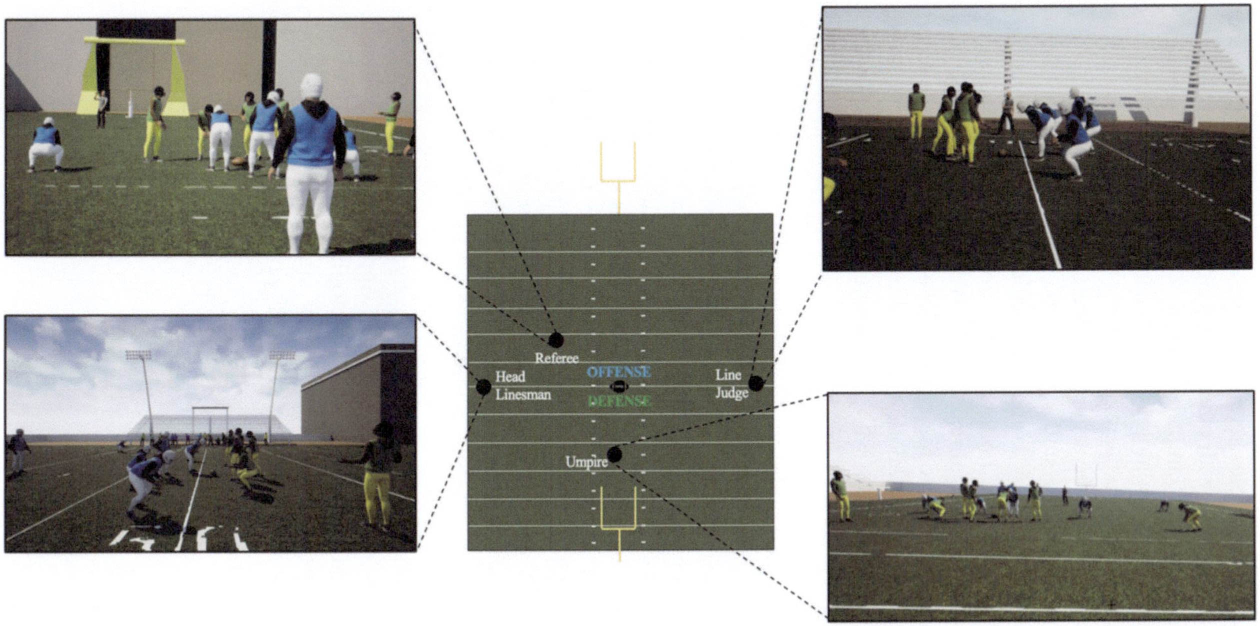

Fig. 9.1 Virtual reality simulation of a play built in Unreal Engine for referee training. The simulation provides training with different angles that can be viewed in real time to provide referees with additional insight into how plays get be better assessed. Referees are able to move around and employ neuro-ophthalmic principles such as field of view and dynamic visual acuity to bridge the gap between watching film and on-field refereeing

9.10 Conclusion

Neuro-ophthalmic principles play a key role in the world of sports, and particularly for NFL officiators. To perform at the highest level, NFL officiators are required to apply various rules quickly to multiple moving players at the same time. The neuro-ophthalmic principles of visual acuity versus dynamic visual acuity, maintaining an optimal visual field, and line of sight are critical for proficient officiating. Understanding of these neuro-ophthalmic principles may help guide upcoming officiators in further optimizing officiating strategies. Further research will be required on how to optimize these parameters, and virtual reality is a promising realm to further improve officiating skills.

Acknowledgments The authors wish to recognize and thank the representatives of the National Football League office of game officials, Walt Anderson and Bret Ayers for their collaboration on this manuscript.

Disclosures Dr. Andrew G. Lee is a consultant for the NFL.

References

1. The Pursuit of Perfection- The History and Evolution of the Officials. National Football League. https://operations.nfl.com/officiating/the-officials/history-of-the-official/. Accessed 10 Dec 2023.
2. Schrager: Missed pass interference call in NFC Championship game was the "worst non-call in the history of the sport." NFL- Good Morning Football. https://www.nfl.com/videos/schrager-missed-pass-interference-call-in-nfc-championship-game-was-the-w-401319. Accessed 23 Dec 2022.
3. Kilgore A. How the Saints-Rams no-call changed the NFL. Washington Post. https://www.washingtonpost.com/sports/2019/09/15/how-saints-rams-no-call-changed-nfl/. Published 15 Sept 2019.
4. Dhoot AS, Koziarz A, Lee Y, Chopra C, Micieli JA. Eye injuries and visor use in the National Football League. Ophthalmology. 2021;128(9):1365–7. https://doi.org/10.1016/j.ophtha.2021.01.027.
5. Court H, McLean G, Guthrie B, Mercer SW, Smith DJ. Visual impairment is associated with physical and mental comorbidities in older adults: a cross-sectional study. BMC Med. 2014;12(1):181. https://doi.org/10.1186/s12916-014-0181-7.
6. Haring RS, Sheffield ID, Canner JK, Schneider EB. Epidemiology of sports-related eye injuries in the United States. JAMA Ophthalmol. 2016;134(12):1382. https://doi.org/10.1001/jamaophthalmol.2016.4253.
7. Patel V, Pakravan P, Mehra D, Watane A, Yannuzzi NA, Sridhar J. Trends in sports-related ocular trauma in United States Emergency Departments from 2010 to 2019: multi-center cross-sectional study. Semin Ophthalmol. 2023;38(4):333–7. https://doi.org/10.1080/08820538.2022.2107400.
8. Miller RA, Rogers RR, Williams TD, et al. Effects of protective american football headgear on peripheral vision reaction time and visual target detection in Division I NCAA football players. Sports. 2019;7(9):213. https://doi.org/10.3390/sports7090213.

9. Edwards JC, Bodle JD. Causes and consequences of sports concussion. J Law Med Ethics. 2014;42(2):128–32. https://doi.org/10.1111/jlme.12126.
10. Mack CD, Solomon G, Covassin T, Theodore N, Cárdenas J, Sills A. Epidemiology of concussion in the National Football League, 2015-2019. Sports Health. 2021;13(5):423–30. https://doi.org/10.1177/19417381211011446.
11. Mack C, Myers E, Barnes R, Solomon G, Sills A. Engaging athletic trainers in concussion detection: overview of the National Football League ATC Spotter Program, 2011–2017. J Athl Train. 2019;54(8):852–7. https://doi.org/10.4085/1062-6050-181-19.
12. Mack C, Sendor RR, Solomon G, et al. Enhancing concussion management in the National Football League: evolution and initial results of the Unaffiliated Neurotrauma Consultants Program, 2012-2017. Neurosurgery. 2020;87(2):312–9. https://doi.org/10.1093/neuros/nyz481.
13. Bailey AM, McMurry TL, Cormier JM, et al. Comparison of laboratory and on-field performance of american football helmets. Ann Biomed Eng. 2020;48(11):2531–41. https://doi.org/10.1007/s10439-020-02627-5.
14. Schalter T. Highlighting the Responsibility of Each NFL Official. Bleacher Report. Published December 13, 2012. https://bleacherreport.com/articles/1443378-highlighting-the-responsibility-of-each-nfl-official. Accessed 27 Jan 2023.
15. NFL Officials: preparing for success. NFL Football Operations. https://operations.nfl.com/officiating/nfl-officials-preparing-for-success/https://operations.nfl.com/officiating/nfl-officials-preparing-for-success/. Accessed 24 Dec 2022.
16. Goodell R. Official playing rules of the National Football League. Published 2022. https://operations.nfl.com/media/5kvgzyss/2022-nfl-rulebook-final.pdf. Accessed 23 Dec 2022.
17. Spector RH. Visual Fields. In: Walker HK, Hall WD, Hurst JW, editors. Clinical methods: the history, physical, and laboratory examinations. 3rd ed. Butterworths; 1990. http://www.ncbi.nlm.nih.gov/books/NBK220/. Accessed 29 Dec 2022.
18. Kedar S, Ghate D, Corbett J. Visual fields in neuro-ophthalmology. Indian J Ophthalmol. 2011;59(2):103. https://doi.org/10.4103/0301-4738.77013.
19. Mosquera SA, Verma S, McAlinden C. Centration axis in refractive surgery. Eye Vis. 2015;2(1):4. https://doi.org/10.1186/s40662-015-0014-6.
20. Quevedo L, Aznar-Casanova JA, Aparecido da Silva J. Dynamic visual acuity. Trends Psychol. 2018;26(3).
21. Waisberg E, Ong J, Paladugu P, et al. Dynamic visual acuity as a biometric for astronaut performance and safety. Life Sci Space Res. 2023;37:3–6. https://doi.org/10.1016/j.lssr.2023.01.002.
22. Mahanama B, Jayawardana Y, Rengarajan S, et al. Eye movement and pupil measures: a review. Front Comput Sci. 2022;3:733531. https://doi.org/10.3389/fcomp.2021.733531.
23. Wong A. The vergence system. In: Eye movement disorders. Oxford University Press; 2008. https://doi.org/10.1093/oso/9780195324266.003.0012.
24. Woods AJ, Kranjec A, Lehet M, Chatterjee A. Expertise and decision-making in American football. Front Psychol. 2015;6:6. https://doi.org/10.3389/fpsyg.2015.00994.
25. Zapetal A. A structured curriculum in neuro-ophthalmic principles for National Football League (NFL) game officials (in press). Presented at: American Academy of Ophthalmology (AAO) 2022 Meeting; 1 October 2022.
26. Ong J, Tavakkoli A, Zaman N, et al. Terrestrial health applications of visual assessment technology and machine learning in spaceflight associated neuro-ocular syndrome. npj Microgravity. 2022;8(1):37. https://doi.org/10.1038/s41526-022-00222-7.
27. Ong J, Zaman N, Kamran SA, et al. A multi-modal visual assessment system for monitoring Spaceflight Associated Neuro-Ocular Syndrome (SANS) during long duration spaceflight. J Vis. 2022;22(3):6. https://doi.org/10.1167/jov.22.3.6.

28. Waisberg E, Ong J, Zaman N, Kamran SA, Lee AG, Tavakkoli A. Head-mounted dynamic visual acuity for G-transition effects during interplanetary spaceflight: technology development and results from an early validation study. Aerosp Med Hum Perform. 2022;93(11):800–5. https://doi.org/10.3357/AMHP.6092.2022.
29. Waisberg E, Ong J, Paladugu P, et al. Advances in machine learning to detect preventable causes of blindness. Eye. 2022; https://doi.org/10.1038/s41433-022-02354-2.
30. Waisberg E, Ong J, Paladugu P, et al. Optimizing screening for preventable blindness with head-mounted visual assessment technology. J Vis Impair Blindness. 2022;116(4):579–81. https://doi.org/10.1177/0145482X221124186.

Chapter 10
Combat Sports in Ophthalmology

Hamza Memon, Nicholas Panzo, Joshua Ong, and Andrew G. Lee

10.1 Introduction

In combat sports, the goal of each participant is to physically defeat their opponent under defined rules of engagement. Combat sports include wrestling, boxing, mixed martial arts (MMA), judo, fencing, and others. The history of combat sports traces back many centuries as demonstrated by cave carvings from 15,000 to 20,000 years ago that illustrate the existence of wrestling, so it is often regarded as the oldest sport [1]. Historically, different traditions have utilized combat sports for various purposes such as conflict dispute, celebration, entertainment, exercise, military

Author, Andrew G. Lee, MD, discloses that he has served or is serving as a consultant for the following companies: AstraZeneca, Alexion, Bristol Mayers Squibb, National Football League, Catalyst, Viridian, Ethyreal, NASA, US Department of Justice, Dompe, and Stoke.

H. Memon (✉) · N. Panzo
Texas A&M School of Engineering Medicine, Houston, TX, USA
e-mail: hamza.memon@tamu.edu

J. Ong
Department of Ophthalmology and Visual Sciences, University of Michigan Kellogg Eye Center, Ann Arbor, MI, USA

A. G. Lee
Department of Ophthalmology, Blanton Eye Institute, Houston Methodist Hospital, Houston, TX, USA

E. Waisberg et al. (eds.), *Ophthalmology of Sports*,
https://doi.org/10.1007/978-3-031-88645-4_10

training, and recreation. Variations of those prehistoric combat sports still exist today and are widely practiced. For example, the Ultimate Fighting Championship (UFC), an event organizer for the sport of MMA, is steadily growing and is estimated to have an annual revenue of $5–6 billion. While the Olympics have showcased combat sports such as boxing and wrestling for over a century, agencies such as the UFC have helped grow their popularity in more recent years.

There are four major categories of combat sports: striking, grappling, weapon usage, and hybrid. Striking sports involve a part of the body rapidly moving towards the opponent with the intention to subdue or incapacitate the opponent. Examples of striking sports include boxing, karate, and taekwondo. Grappling sports, such as wrestling, Jujutsu, and Kung Fu, focus on ground fighting, sweeps, throws, and submission holds. Hybrid combat sports use techniques and theories from multiple other categories. MMA is one of the most popular combat sports in modern times. The last category of combat sports is weapon sports such as fencing, where opponents wield swords. Combat sports are extremely physically demanding and require both physical and cognitive skills. Strength, endurance, speed, agility, coordination, flexibility, and balance are all necessary in combat sports. Injuries are common in combat sports and can result in bodily damage, both temporary or permanent, and, in rare cases, even death.

Injuries in combat sports typically result from striking (e.g., punches and kicks), grappling, or falling. The specific cause of injury varies depending on the type of combat sport. For example, in boxing, the majority of the injuries are to the head, while in judo and wrestling, joints are more likely to be injured [2, 3]. Still, concussions are the most common injuries in combat sports, with one study estimating over half of professional boxing injuries are concussions [4]. To reduce the risk of serious harm, opponents in many combat sports are placed in the same skill category and may be further divided by weight. Although combat sports affect many different body systems, visual injuries are crucial to study and understand.

Vision is essential to athletes because it allows them to perceive, understand, and predict the movement of their opponents. Literature strongly suggests that highly skilled athletes have efficient patterns of visual search compared to athletes with lesser skills [5]. Athletes spend years developing their skills and coordination through their acute senses of perception and cognition. Perception is the detection and interpretation of the various energy forms from one's surroundings [6]. In combat sports, this translates to the visual processing of the opponent's body positioning, head movement, eye movement, and other subtle muscle movements that precede a strike. The ability for an athlete to recognize and respond to their opponent's intended action provides them with a significant advantage to both cause and avoid damage. As technology advances, more and more research is being done to study the visual system in athletes.

10.2 Wrestling

10.2.1 Rules

Wrestling consists of two opponents that grapple to throw or pin their opponents' shoulders on the ground or in the absence of a pin to outscore each other. There are many different versions of wrestling, and each varies slightly depending on the region and culture in which it is practiced. To maintain consistency and standardization in global competitions, the United World Wrestling (UWW) serves as the paramount international governing body, overseeing the organization of both the Olympics and the Wrestling World Championships. Each wrestling match in the Olympics consists of three rounds of two minutes each, totaling six minutes of wrestling time with a 30 second break between each round. A referee is present on the wrestling platform to enforce the rules to ensure safety and fairness. For more equitable competition, competitors are grouped into specific weight categories that are established and regulated by governing bodies like the UWW. Multiple judges oversee each match, evaluating and assigning points to the competitors. Wrestling matches unfold on a square mat, featuring a central circular wrestling zone (depicted in Fig. 10.1). This central area serves as the designated battleground within which the wrestlers must remain during the course of their bout. The orange circle, the passivity zone, represents out of bounds and if the player continuously enters the passivity zone, then they are penalized.

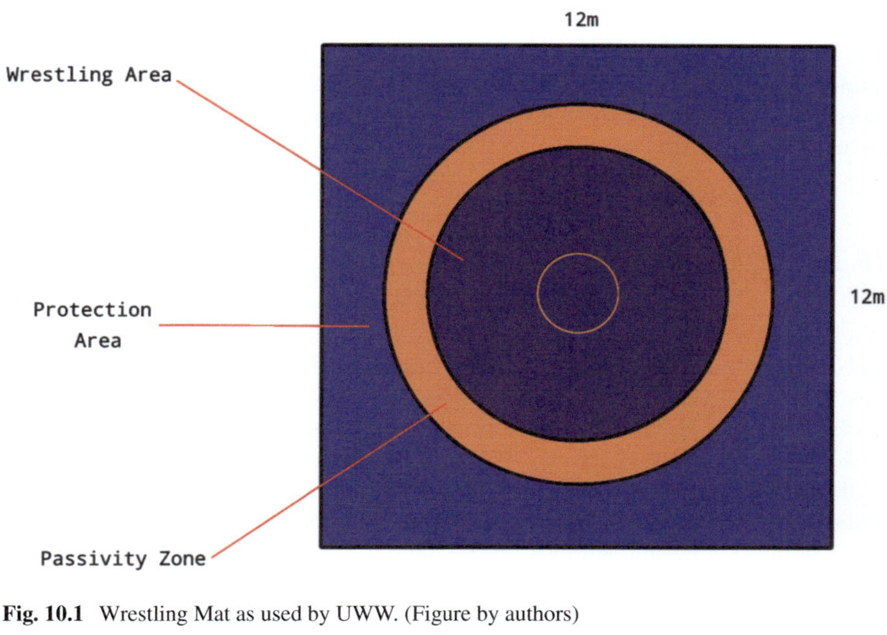

Fig. 10.1 Wrestling Mat as used by UWW. (Figure by authors)

In freestyle wrestling, participants can use their arms and legs to bring down opponents and points are awarded based on throws, holds, takedowns, executing reversals, or pinning the shoulders of the opponent on the ground. Reversal, as the name suggests, is the act of gaining control by negating the advantageous position of the opponent. In addition, between one to five points are awarded based on the move's difficulty (e.g., arching throws). Illegal holds and other negative moves can result in points to the opponent and a caution to the player committing the infraction—the player is disqualified after three cautions. Illegal moves include choking, twisting arms, biting, striking with elbow or knee, and holds or strikes that have a potential to cause injuries to head, neck, or back.

There are four ways to win in an Olympic wrestling match. First, at the end of six minutes, the participant with the most points is declared the winner. If there is a tie, the wrestler that obtained the most points from a single move is declared as the winner. Second, "victory by technical" is declared when a participant has at least a ten-point lead, even if there is time left in the match. Third, a wrestler can win by pinning their opponent's shoulder on the ground long enough to show control of the move. Finally, the fourth way to win is if a player is disqualified because of an illegal move.

Wrestling requires many cognitive and physical skills. Although each wrestling match only lasts six minutes, the match requires cardiovascular, muscular, and mental endurance. Endurance comes in different forms: cardiovascular, muscular, and mental. Cardiovascular endurance is developed with exercises such as running and cycling, muscular endurance is developed with strength training, and mental endurance is necessary to predict and adapt to the opponent while maintaining focus and handling pressure in high stakes situations. All these forms of endurance must work synchronously to obtain maximal output. Other skills such as flexibility, technique, and agility take years and consistent hard work to develop. A final key aspect of training is weight management. Because wrestlers compete within a specific weight category, it is essential they meet the weight requirements while still maximizing endurance, agility, and strength.

10.2.2 Epidemiology

Wrestling is a physical sport that involves complex moves to subdue the opponent, and due to the nature of the sport, it is unsurprising there is a high potential for injuries. Over a six year period, one study found there were over 165,000 emergency department (ED) visits for wrestlers between the ages of 7 and 17 [7]. Fortunately, 97% of the visits were minor and 75% of the injuries occurred above the waist [7]. College wrestling injuries are reported to occur at a rate of 9.6 injuries per 1000 athlete-exposure (athlete's participation in competition where they are exposed to being injured) [8]. Although most of the injuries were minor, 6.3% of the injuries required surgical intervention. The most common location of injuries in wrestling are the knees, shoulders, and ankles with sprains, strains, contusions being the most common type of injuries [8]. Over the years, the average number of injuries reported has increased, which can be attributed to the increase in popularity and participation of the sport [9]. As more research and studies are published, rules and regulations of wrestling have evolved to mitigate the risk of injury, including the establishment of illegal moves and holds.

While ocular injuries are infrequent in wrestling, they do occasionally occur. Collegiate wrestlers have a prevalence of 1 to 2 ocular injuries that occur per season for a team of 25 athletes [10]. Ocular injuries are the least common of the cranio-maxillofacial injuries in wrestlers [9]. Some of the injuries suffered by wrestlers include laceration to the cornea and eyelid, abrasion of eye and conjunctiva, and contusion of the eye. Eyebrow and eyelid contusions are uncommon and represent 1% of injuries while lacerations occur at a higher rate of 2.7%. Orbit injuries are more common than the external eye injuries with eye abrasions occurring at a rate of 4%, eye contusions at 11%, and lacerations at 5% [10].

While most ocular injuries are minor, it is important to know that serious ophthalmic injuries do occur. A 19-year-old wrestler was accidentally elbowed in the eye during a wrestling match, which caused eye lacerations and orbital blow-out fracture. An orbital blow-out fracture is caused by a high impact to the eye, increasing the intraorbital hydraulic pressure and causing fracture of the wall or floor of the orbit. In a similar case, a 20-year-old college wrestler accidentally struck his eye on his knee when thrown by the opponent which also caused an orbital blow-out fracture. The classic symptoms of this kind of fracture include enophthalmos (sunken globe), diplopia when looking upward outward, and numbing of the infraorbital nerve. In both instances, the wrestlers were sent to the emergency room for immediate care. In some cases, surgery is required [11]. When severe, orbital fractures can require surgical intervention to restore vision and avoid long-term complications. Fortunately, neither of these wrestlers required surgery and both eventually fully recovered [11].

Besides blunt force trauma and laceration, other ocular pathologies have been reported in wrestling. Close contact sports such as wrestling provide an ideal environment for transmission of microorganisms. In 1989, 145 high school wrestlers participated in a multi week wrestling camp which resulted in an outbreak of Human Simplex Virus 1 (HSV-1) [12]. Ocular clinical manifestations of HSV-1 include keratitis, conjunctivitis, and uveitis. Proper management of HSV-1 ocular manifestations can prevent complications and preserve vision. This outbreak is an example that highlights the potential of transmission of microorganisms that can cause severe pathologies. Another reported ophthalmic injury is keratoconus. A 30-year-old with a 14-year history of wrestling had gradual progressive vision loss bilaterally, as well as a decrease in visual acuity. A corneal topography study confirmed the diagnosis of keratoconus. A similar case was reported in a wrestler with a 20-year history in the sport. Wrestlers are repeatedly involved in moves that increase the intraocular pressure which can push the cornea outward. The outward push alters the shape of the cornea and cause vision problems like blurry vision [13]. Keratoconus can usually be treated with contact lenses or, in severe cases, surgery.

10.2.3 Equipment

Wrestling equipment requirements vary based on the level of competition. Wrestlers wear a tightly fitted, single piece suit without any rough edges called a singlet. Wrestlers also wear shoes that allow mobility and grip on the wrestling pad and light knee pads, if allowed. Headgear and ear protections are permitted in intercollegiate and grade school wrestling; however, it may be optional or prohibited in adult competitions. Wrestlers are not allowed to wear any jewelry or any bandages that are not approved by the medical staff. Again, depending on the competition, mouth guards are sometimes optional and other times required. Wrestling goggles do exist, and while they could help prevent ocular injuries, they are not widely adopted nor allowed in competitions. Other eye protection is generally not utilized to avoid any potential advantages or disadvantages to eyesight. As is, the most widely implemented ocular protection is the wrestling rules placed by the governing body, such as prohibition of eye poking.

10.3 Boxing

Boxing is one of the oldest sports known to mankind. The earliest evidence of boxing dates back to Mesopotamia around the 4th millennium BC [14]. The history of boxing is rich with traditional, political, cultural, entertainment, and recreational values that shape its modern form. In the early years, boxing was a sport available to all social classes; however, most participants were from distinguished backgrounds. Today, many people would consider boxing a brutal sport. That said, when compared to the early days of boxing, today's boxing is much safer and better regulated. For example, early participants would only occasionally use gloves. The Greeks used training gloves similar to modern gloves, but only during training. Even more, other cultures weaponized gloves: the Romans wore gloves with embedded metal or spikes to cause harm to the opponent. In fact, some boxing matches would be fought until one of the contestants died from their injuries. Boxing was also used to train military personnel on combat techniques and strength.

10.3.1 Rules

Rules and regulations of each sport are designed to decrease the risk factors that can cause serious bodily harm to the participants. Boxing without gloves, boxing against different weight classes, and executing certain moves are all illegal today [14]. Rules of boxing slightly differ based on the governing group that organized the event, but this chapter will focus on the rules implemented for the Olympic boxing games. Each boxing game consists of two fighters that will box against each other with a referee in the ring. The objective of the game is to "hit and not get hit" or, in more elaborate terms, to incapacitate the opponent by striking the head or the torso.

The fight takes place on an elevated square ring that is approximately 8 meters on each side. Boxers today use gloves that are either 12 oz, 14 oz, or 16 oz. The use of padded gloves further protects fighters from causing injuries to themselves or their opponent. Similar to wrestling, boxers are segregated based on their weight, but boxers are able to fight in different weight classes as long as they meet the requirement of that weight class. In the Olympics, each boxing match consists of three rounds of three minutes each with a one-minute break in between.

The referee in the ring serves to ensure fairness, to start and stop fights, and to moderate other aspects of the match. In addition, there are multiple judges who sit outside the ring to keep track of the score throughout the fight. The score is calculated based on strikes to target areas (head, face, torso), technique, and tactical superiority. If there is any illegal contact or other infringement, deductions can be made to the score. A foul in boxing is defined as any strike or movement that is not permitted and is classified as either intentional or accidental. As the names suggest, intentional fouls are those the opponent knowingly committed while accidental fouls are those that occur inadvertently. When the boxer commits an intentional foul that results in a severe injury, the boxer is immediately disqualified. On the other hand, if the injury is not severe and the match can continue, the boxer committing the foul will have points deducted from the score sheet. However, if the match does continue despite the injury and then terminated in a later round due to that injury, there are two possible scenarios: (1) if the injured boxer has more points at the time of termination, then that boxer is declared the winner; (2) if the injured boxer has less or equal points, then the match is declared a draw. If an accidental foul occurs resulting in an injury severe enough to stop the match before round 4, then the match will be declared as "no decision." However, if the injury occurs after round 4, then the player that has more points at the time of termination of the match will be declared the winner.

Any strikes that are not delivered from the boxer's gloves (e.g. legs, head, shoulder, arms) are considered a foul. Pushing the opponent is considered a foul because it leads to an unfair advantage. Attacking the opponent when they are down or knocked out could result in a penalty or disqualification. Other unsportsman-like conduct such as talking, biting, assaulting the referee or any action that is beyond the realm of acceptable movements are prohibited. Boxers are required to wear a mouthpiece at all times while they engage in a fight. Intentional removal of the mouthpiece during the fight could also result in a penalty. The rules of the game are enforced to ensure maximal safety of the participants as well as the referee.

Despite the perceived simplicity of the sport, there are multiple avenues for victory. The score is calculated at the end to determine which participant has won the fight. The first way to win is by points, in which ringside judges determine the number of points each player has at the end of the match. If all judges agree on a winner, it is called a unanimous decision. However, if all judges do not agree on a winner, the decision of the majority of the judges prevails and it is called a "split decision." A game can be declared a draw if all or even the majority of judges agree. Another way to win is by technical knockout (TKO), which is when the participant or their team stops the fight for any reason or if the participant cannot continue after the break between rounds. Similarly, technical knockout injury (TKO-I) is when the referee determines that a participant is not fit due to sustained injury. When a player is knocked down, the referee will count until ten and if the boxer is unable to get up, then the opponent is declared as the winner by knockout (KO). As previously mentioned, there are many fouls that can result in disqualification which then awards the victory to the opposing player. If a player does not appear for the fight, the opponent is declared as victorious by "win by walkover." In rare circumstances, a game may be declared "no contest" due to events outside the control of the participants or referee that prevent the fight from happening (e.g., venue problems or damaged boxing ring).

10.3.2 Epidemiology

Boxing is a dangerous sport because of its objective of incapacitating the opponent. The strikes generate tremendous force that has the potential to cause significant damage to the opponent or even death. Frequent blows to the head have rendered fatalities, a not uncommon occurrence in boxing. According to CNN, an average of 13 boxers succumb annually to injuries sustained during matches, and nearly 2000 deaths have been recorded since 1890 as a result of injuries sustained during boxing matches. A recent example is of a South African boxer named Simiso Buthelezi who died due to an intracranial bleed acquired during a boxing match. Unfortunately, most of the studies of injuries in boxing are retrospective and were done decades ago [2, 15].

The most effective way to acquire points in boxing is to intentionally make contact with the opponent's face or head. As a result, head and face injuries make up about 70% of injuries obtained during a match and about 30% of injuries obtained in training [16]. There has been an increasing interest in researching and evaluating long-term neurodegenerative effects on boxers, especially those caused by intracranial injuries [15]. Boxers who received a significant number of strikes to the head were more likely to experience long-term neurologic disability such as dementia pugilistica [17]. Additionally, these repeated strikes to the head can result in damages to the brain, oculomotor, and vestibular systems [15, 16]. Other common injuries in boxing include lacerations to the face, eyes, damage to teeth, and cervical spinal column damage [15]. A study investigating boxing-related injuries revealed there are over 8500 annual visits to US emergency departments for such injuries between 1990 and 2008 (Fig. 10.2) [18]. The most common diagnosis in the ED was fracture, soft tissue injury, and head injury (mostly concussion) [18]. Later outcomes of concussions include impairment of the vestibular and oculomotor systems which can present with vertigo, dizziness, blurred vision, diplopia, and headaches. Even though an athlete may recover from a concussion and return to fighting, the repeated blows to the head leave a lasting impact. A recent study indicates that

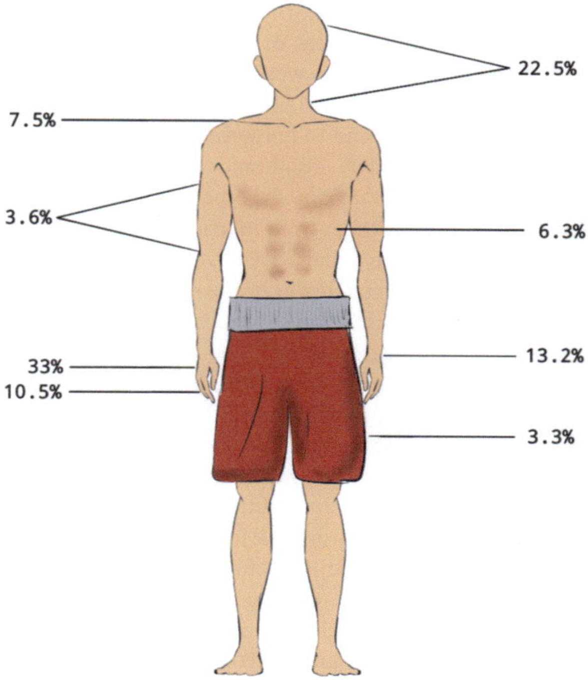

Fig. 10.2 Body region boxing injuries presented to the emergency department between 1990 and 2008. (Figure by authors). Head and Neck: 22.5%; Shoulder: 7.5%; Torso: 6.3%; Arm and Elbow: 3.6%; Wrist: 13.2%; Hand: 33%; Finger: 10.5%; Lower Limb: 3.3%; Other: 0.1%

repeated head blows are correlated with delayed muscular response and negatively correlated with latency amplitude [19].

Boxing has one of the higher rates of injuries at 17–25 per 100 professional male fights. However, female boxing seems to be safer compared to males—male boxers are more likely (3.6 per 100 boxer-rounds) to sustain injuries as opposed to female boxers (1.2 per 100 boxer-rounds). Additionally, male boxers have a knockout rate that is 5 times higher than female boxers [17].

Medical councils around the world have led movements to ban boxing because of these acute and chronic injuries. It is estimated that 27% to 93% of boxing injuries are to the head which can cause neurologic injuries [2]. One of the main targets for boxers is the head because they cause the most damage and increase the possibility of knockouts, they are one of the main targets. Strikes to the head or face can cause facial lacerations and injuries to the nose, mouth, jaw, and eyes [17]. The most common injury site for the head is the eye, eyelid, and eyebrow region, accounting for almost half of the injuries [2]. In fact, boxing accounts for a quarter of severe eye injuries worldwide because the eye is exposed without any safety equipment [20]. As a result, ringside medical staff continuously monitor the boxer's ocular system.

Periorbital ecchymosis and eyelid lacerations are common injuries that can be diagnosed at ringside. More serious injuries are often a challenge to diagnose due to the lack of pupil dilation or boxers hiding their injury in order to prevent the match termination. Ocular trauma in boxing is so common that a study found that 66% to

76% of boxers had signs of asymptomatic ocular trauma [21]. Eye examinations revealed structural changes of the retina, iris, lens, and orbital arch [22]. On the other hand, 68% of boxers were found to have vision-threatening damage, which, in this study, is classified as significant damage to the retina, the lens, or macula [23].

Boxing can also lead to numerous ocular injuries in the anterior chamber of the eye. One of the most common and undiagnosed injuries is corneal abrasions, because of its low morbidity. Another possible injury is hyphema, which is bleeding into the anterior chamber from injuries to the iris or surrounding structures. Damage to lenses and change in capacity have also been reported in boxers. There is a 6% to 22% incidence of cataracts in professional boxing [22, 24]. The most common type of cataract in boxers is the subscapular posterior cataract [21, 23]. Cataracts may present asymptomatic until the opacity alterations increase blurry vision. Other injuries related to the lens include the possibility of lens dislocation which has a reported incidence of about 7% [25]. Trauma, in this case a punch, is the most common way to rupture the zonules that hold the lens in place. Other anterior chamber injuries such as subconjunctival hemorrhage, iritis, cyclodialysis, and iridodialysis are possible in boxing. In addition to the anterior segment injuries, posterior segment injuries are also prevalent in boxing.

Posterior segment injuries to the eye include damage to the vitreous humor, retina, choroid, and the optic nerve. One of the most common and severe ocular injuries in boxing is traumatic rhegmatogenous retinal detachment which occurs when the retina is separated from the surrounding connecting tissue. Wills Eye Hospital reported treating 9 boxers that had retina injury, 8 of whom had retinal detachment and a large tear in the retina without any symptoms [26]. The true incidence of retinal tears is unclear, with reports placing them between 1 and 24% of all ocular injuries. Some boxers have even suffered from bilateral retina detachments, albeit less than 2% [23, 25]. Despite the varying incidence rates reported of retinal detachment, it is imperative that physicians observe boxers for potential retina pathologies.

Besides retinal detachment, other posterior segment injuries, such as macular pathologies, may occur in boxing. The macula is responsible for the central vision of the eye and contains the highest density of cones (color sensory cells). Macular abnormalities are not common in boxers with an incidence rate of 8% [23]. In addition, blunt force trauma from a boxing punch can fracture the bone surrounding the eye, possibly resulting in the compression of the optic nerve by the fragmented bone, called optic neuropathy. Another common ocular pathology in boxers, similar to wrestlers, is the orbital blowout fracture. A study analyzing the occurrence of 1141 orbital fracture in the US Army reported that one of the major causes of orbital blowout fracture is fighting [27].

A rare occurrence of left central retinal artery occlusion (CRAO) was reported when a 21-year-old boxer was punched in the neck which caused a carotid artery dissection [28]. CRAO is a serious condition in which the artery supplying the retina is occluded, resulting in sudden, painless vision loss. CRAO is considered a medical emergency that requires immediate attention from an ophthalmologist to attempt to restore vision. This case is an excellent example of the unpredictable injuries and the mechanism by which they can occur in boxing.

10.3.3 Equipment

Similar to wrestling, boxing equipment varies based on the competition and governing body. The most effective protection for boxers are the rules and regulations. In the 2024 Olympics, for example, boxers are required to wear padded gloves that enclose their entire hand. The weight of the glove is strictly regulated and inspected by the officials. Hand wraps must be worn to protect their hands and wrists. Only female boxers are allowed to wear a head guard. Shorts, skirts, and vests for females are acceptable attire during a match. Mouthguards must be worn at all times during a match; if a mouth guard is removed, the match will be stopped by the referee. Shoes without spikes and heels must be worn. Groin protectors must be worn by males, but it is optional for females to wear. Breast protectors are optional for females. Ocular protection is often not utilized in competitive boxing; however, recreational boxers occasionally use goggles or headgear. There is a possibility that safety goggles may increase the risk of orbital fracture due to the force distribution; thus, head gear that protect the periorbital region may help mitigate the risk of ocular injuries.

10.4 Mixed Martial Arts

Mixed Martial Arts (MMA) is a full-contact combat sport that includes aspects of wrestling, boxing, Muay Thai, and Brazilian Jiu Jitsu. MMA is one of the fastest growing sports globally because of media coverage and marketing organizations such as UFC. The birth of MMA can be traced back to 649 BC when the sport pankration was included in the Olympics. Pankration is a Greek word that combines two words "pan," meaning "all," and "kration," meaning "powers." Pankration consisted of elements of boxing and wrestling [29]. However, modern MMA was officially born in November of 1993 during the inaugural UFC fight. In the early years, very few rules existed which allowed fighters from various backgrounds to face each other. Lack of rules paved the way for frequent mismatched opponents and a multitude of medical disasters. Medical aspects aside, these mismatches made for very exciting and entertaining fights for the audiences and ultimately played a significant role in attracting a fan base.

Due to the aggressiveness of the fights and the brutal bouts with a lack of a mature organizing body, MMA was initially banned in most of the United States. There were only three rules—no biting, eye gouging, and groin kicks—UFC was heavily promoted as "there are no rules" to provide the audience an experience that mimics a raw street fight. Accordingly, the violent nature of the sport invited a flood of concern from medical associations including the American Medical Association, Canadian Medical Association, and Australian Medical Association [30]. In the early 2000s, MMA restructured with more rules under a new ownership of UFC, which allowed the sport to grow more prominent in the United States. Still, MMA is a relatively new sport, so the research is still limited.

10.4.1 Rules

In the early years, UFC experienced scrutiny by politicians, medical community, media, and sports organizations. In 2001, Zuffa LLC purchased UFC and redesigned the sport to reverse the controversy and expand the sport. UFC went from having only 3 rules to having over 30 rules and establishing weight classes to ensure participant safety. The rules listed in this chapter will consist of the largest promoting organization, the UFC, though other international promoting organizations have their own variation of rules. The main objective of MMA is similar to wrestling and boxing—to defeat the opponent. However, unlike wrestling and boxing which limits fighters to only one technique, MMA is a combination of various fighting techniques.

MMA fights are violent and can easily cause permanent injury to the participants. In fact, because of the violent nature of the fights, bleeding during the fight is not uncommon. Pre-fight protocol requires medical examinations to assess the fighters' physical health for their safety and the safety of their opponents. MMA is a full contact sport; thus, the fighters are in close proximity to each other. Contagious diseases such as Hepatitis B, C, and HIV are usually tested as part of the medical exam, and a full physical exam is performed by a physician. Cardiovascular exams and reports are also part of the medical exams, and, if the ringside physician finds them to be necessary, radiological exams are also completed. For female fighters, a negative pregnancy test is also required. In some states, a neurological exam is necessary for everyone, while other states require one only for fighters of a certain age or fighters that have accumulated a certain number of fights. Neurological examinations determine whether any brain damage is present, which is quite common for a sport that is focused on causing as much damage to the opponent as possible. Ophthalmic exams are sometimes required as well to determine if any visual problems exist. Medical exams play a critical role in keeping everyone involved, especially the fighters, safe. The exams also prevent the sport from getting a bad reputation should a pre-existing health issue manifest in front of the audience.

Similar to boxing and wrestling, MMA is a contest between two human fighters. The fight is held in an 8-sided platform which is now commonly referred to as an octagon. During the fight, there are two fighters in the octagon as well as a referee. The referee plays a similar role as the other combat sports discussed in this chapter—to ensure fighter safety while adhering to the rules. The referee is the only person allowed to stop the fight. In the UFC, non-championship matches consist of 3 rounds while championship or main events are 5 rounds. Each round is 5 minutes long with a 1-minute break in between each round. Fighters are placed into one of the 14 weight categories to ensure fair and safe competition, similar to boxing and wrestling. The only protective attire the players are allowed to wear are gloves and a mouthpiece.

Fouls are an essential part of regulating the game. The use of the head as an instrument to strike is considered illegal. Eye gouging is strictly prohibited; however, direct blows to the orbital regions are acceptable. The use of fingers to hook into the opponents' eyes, nose, mouth, or any other area causing stretching of the skin is prohibited. Any strikes to the spine or the back of the head (crown of the head to the occipital region) are illegal. Downward pointing linear elbow strikes are against the rules. When a player is grounded (any part of the body besides a single hand and soles of foot are touching the fighting area), kneeing or kicking the head are unacceptable. Stomping the opponent which consists of striking with the bottom of the feet while bending at the knee is considered illegal. A fighter is not allowed to hold onto the gloves or shorts of the opponent to gain control. Poking the opponent in any orifice or laceration is prohibited. Unsportsmanlike conduct, ignoring the referee, and use of offensive language during the fight is not allowed. Attacking the opponent after the round has ended or after the bell are strictly prohibited. Attacking the referee or the opponent while under the care of the referee is not allowed. Any interference from the team of the opponent is not acceptable. Fouls can result in point deductions for the aggressor or even disqualification.

Each match is judged by a minimum of three ringside judges and adheres to a 10-point system. This point system dictates that at the end of each round, the winner must be awarded 10 points, while the loser is awarded 9 or less points. In rare circumstances, both players can be awarded 10 points. Judges assess various MMA techniques, like striking and grappling, effectiveness, and control of the fight. Effective striking is rewarded based on the impact of strike and effective grappling is based on effective takedowns, submissions attempts, and reversals. There are multiple ways by which a fighter can be granted victory, one of which is to win by submission. Submission includes "tap out," where the opponent uses their body to indicate to the referee that they no longer wish to continue the fight. Verbal tap out is using words rather than a physical motion to indicate the desire to terminate the fight. Technical submission is when the opponent is rendered unconscious or severely injured. Tap out, verbal tap out, and technical submission are all considered wins by submission. Technical knockout is classified as a stoppage of the contest for two reasons: (1) the opponent can no longer defend themselves and (2) medical stoppage due to injury. Win by knockout is when a contestant is rendered unconscious or unable to defend because of a strike by the opponent. Win by disqualification is when the contestant has committed multiple fouls or caused a match-ending injury from an intentional foul. No contest is when the contest is terminated prematurely without finishing enough rounds to warrant a score. Decisions are similar to boxing; they can be unanimous, split, majority, or technical.

10.4.2 Epidemiology

MMA is an extreme sport that is filled with violence and aggression. Some even consider it the most violent sport. While MMA is a regulated and organized sport that has rules to protect the fighters, the inherent nature of the sport produces many injuries. MMA is thought to have similar injury patterns to other combat sports (i.e., boxing, wrestling, kickboxing), but the patterns in MMA are more pronounced because it combines all the individual combat sports. Fighters deliver numerous powerful strikes in the form of punches, elbow strikes, kicks, knees, take downs, chokes, and joint locks, all which can cause significant damage. Although MMA involves different fighting styles, and it has 65% more injuries than boxing, the rate of concussion in MMA is less than that of boxing [31]. This is understandable because the target area in boxing is primarily strikes to the head while MMA also includes non-strike moves such as grappling and takedowns. The most common type of injuries in MMA is reported to be face laceration followed by hand fractures [31]. Periocular lacerations are the most common type of face laceration that can cause a fight to end [32]. Head strikes are the most common way of causing a knockout and the most common location to be struck is the mandible, comprising over half of the strike location (Fig. 10.3) [33].

Stopping fights due to injury is a common occurrence in MMA; over 70% of fights are stopped as a result of injuries. One study reported an average of 48.3 concussions per 1000 fights, which is more than twice the concussion rate in kickboxing [32].This number is possibly even higher due to a lack of rigorous research and potential underreporting from the fighters. As a consequence of concussions, MMA athletes have been found to have impaired vestibulo-ocular reflex [34]. Besides head injuries, lower and upper extremity injuries make up the majority of the injuries. In a sport like MMA, in which various techniques are utilized, a wide variety of injuries occur including contusions, fractures, dislocations, joint trauma, sprains, and strains [35].

The ocular system is prone to trauma due to its anatomical location which coincides with one of the common target areas in combat sports. Limited studies have evaluated the occurrence of ocular injury in MMA, but the prevalence of ocular

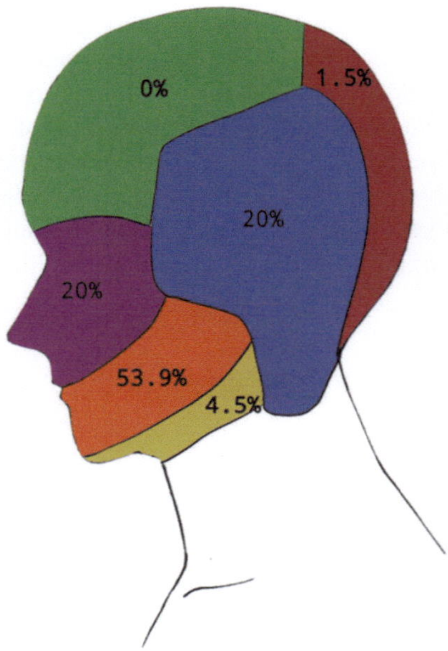

Fig. 10.3 Diagram of a human head in profile view, divided into colored sections with percentages for knock out strike location. The top of the head is green with 0%, the midface is purple with 20%, the side of the head is blue with 20%, the back of the head is maroon with 1.5%, the cheek is orange with 53.9%, and the jaw is brown with 4.5%

injuries in MMA could be between 5.8% and 8.3%, [35–37] while the annual rate of eye injuries per 100 fights was determined to range between 2.56% and 12.22%. The most common injuries include eyebrow and eyelid lacerations, eye lacerations, and orbital fracture, and less common injuries include those to the retina and corneal abrasions [36]. Since the ocular system plays a crucial role in MMA sports, it is no surprise that ocular injuries interfere with optimal performance. Over two-thirds of fighters who suffer from an ocular injury end up losing the fight [36].

Eyebrow and eyelid lacerations constitute the majority of ocular injuries, accounting for 43% of all such injuries, while corneal abrasions account for only 1% of ocular injuries in MMA [36]. Corneal abrasions are defined as a scratch to the surface of the cornea. In the general population, corneal abrasions are a more common occurrence as they make up almost half of all ocular-related emergency room visits [38]. In fact, cornea is so fragile that abrasions can be caused by contact lenses or fingernails. Corneal abrasions have a quick recovery and mild symptoms, so fighters are likely to not report such injuries. As a result, the documented number is likely much lower than the actual rate.

Severe laceration and abrasions have the potential to cause irreversible damage to vision. Other high potential ocular injuries in MMA include orbital fractures and retinal detachments. Orbital fractures are seen in other combat sports such as wrestling and boxing. Orbital fractures, also known as "blowout" fractures, make up 17% of all ocular injuries sustained in MMA [36]. Blowout fractures are a result of blunt force trauma to the periocular region, particularly on the globe. Posterior segment injuries such as retinal injuries are infrequent in MMA compared to other injuries as they account for 3% of orbital injuries [39]. Former UFC star Michael Bisping was on the receiving end of a kick to the head that resulted in blindness in his right eye. In 2013, Bisping suffered from retinal detachment that resulted in vision loss. For months, Bisping kept the injury to himself to avoid being sidelined by the medical staff. Eventually, his symptoms progressed and despite several surgeries, his vision could not be restored.

10.4.3 Equipment

In UFC, male fighters are required to wear shorts and no top while females wear shorts and tops. Fighters may wrap their hands with soft gauze, no longer than 15 yards, distributed evenly on each hand. Fighters are required to wear a mouthguard at all times during a fight. If the mouthpiece is ejected, the referee will pause the match until it is cleaned and re-worn. Gloves must be worn by the contestants during the match. The gloves for MMA are different from those used in boxing, MMA gloves are lighter and smaller with less padding and do not completely cover the fingers. There is no indication of use of protective eye equipment in MMA. Despite rules to prevent eye poking and gauging, accidental injuries do occur to the fighters. A recent example is Justin Tafa getting poked in his eye, which resulted in the termination of the fight.

10.5 Injuries in Combat Sports

The anatomy of the orbit is designed to minimize injuries to the eye. The eye sits in a socket, surrounded by bones that provide support and structure, and is surrounded by a pad of fat. This padding, which also lacks any firm attachments, allows for force absorption. In addition, the blink reflex is an essential form of protection that reduces damage such as abrasions. Despite the protective anatomical design of the orbital, ocular injuries are common. Unfortunately, many injuries can be attributed to the lack of protective ocular gear in combat sports.

Due to the lack of ocular protection, the eye is frequently exposed to the large forces from punches or kicks. The force delivered from a punch of a professional boxer can reach up to 5358 Newtons (N), which greatly exceeds the force necessary to create an eye contusion [40].

There are two general mechanisms by which ocular injury occurs in boxing: coup and contrecoup. While more frequently used to describe brain injuries, these mechanisms can also describe injury to the eye. Coup is an injury resulting from direct contact with a blunt force and includes external injuries such as lid laceration and corneal abrasions. Contrecoup is an injury caused by the shock waves from blunt force that transverse the region of impact. Injuries caused by the contrecoup mechanism include macular holes, cataracts, and superonasal retinal dialysis [41].

10.5.1 Eyebrow and Eyelid Lacerations

Eyelid and eyebrow lacerations can quite easily occur in combat sports by various movements such as getting punched, kicked, taken down, or accidentally jabbed. Eyebrow and eyelid lacerations are cuts or tears to the eyelid or the eyebrow. The cuts can be superficial or deep and can include the soft tissues surrounding it. These lacerations can cause bruising, bleeding, or swelling which can all interfere with vision. Athletes that present with any such lacerations should be subjected to further ocular examination, especially given the proximity of injury to other ocular structures. A slit lamp examination must be conducted for the anterior segment as well as posterior segment imaging in patients who have sustained an ocular fight injury.

Often, lacerations that are cleaned will heal on their own, but if the laceration is deep enough, it may require sutures. In rare cases, reconstructive surgery is required especially when a large soft tissue defect exists [42]. If surrounding structures or glands are damaged, then further treatment may be required. To prevent infection to the laceration, antibiotics are typically prescribed.

10.5.2 Hyphema

Hyphema refers to the accumulation of blood in the anterior chamber of the eye. Hyphema can occur spontaneously by hematological pathologies (e.g., leukemia, von Willebrand disease and hemophilia), but one of the common causes is trauma. Vision-threatening complications of hyphema include increased intraocular pressure, secondary hemorrhage, optic atrophy, and accommodation impairment [43]. Although hyphema often occurs as a result of trauma in fighters, other causes must be ruled out. Hyphema can indicate the presence of major ocular or surrounding tissue injuries which can be challenging to identify [44]. Hyphema is commonly diagnosed using a slit lamp biomicroscope, although in cases of significant hyphema, a simple pen light can be adequate for initial diagnosis. Hyphema can be categorized into four categories: [44]

- Grade I: Blood covers one-third of the anterior chamber.
- Grade II: Blood covers one-third to one-half of the anterior chamber.
- Grade III: Blood covers one-half to less than the entire anterior chamber.
- Grade IV: Total clotted blood.

Management of hyphema can include a pharmacological approach through the use of cycloplegics, steroids, anti-glaucoma, and analgesics [43]. Athletes are also provided with an eye-shield to limit activity and prevent further damage. The affected eye is observed for a few days for re-bleeds or other complications but, in most cases, pharmacological treatment provides a complete recovery. In cases where medication is ineffective or complications arise, surgical intervention is required. Surgeries remove blood from the chamber and correct any other complications.

10.5.3 Corneal Abrasions

Failure to accurately diagnose and appropriately manage corneal abrasions can lead to serious threats to vision. In combat sports, corneal abrasions can be easily acquired by corneal contact with a glove, fighting surface, any other body part of the opponent. Corneal abrasions are a result of scratches or cuts to the anterior portion of the ocular epithelium [41, 45]. The symptoms include redness, pain, light sensitivity, and discomfort. A detailed and complete exam is necessary for someone presenting with a potential corneal abrasion. Because the cornea is a clear membrane, it can be challenging to see the abrasions; thus, a fluorescein dye is used to visualize the abrasions under cobalt blue light. Most corneal abrasions recover within 2–3 days; however, some can cause vision-threatening complications if not adequately treated [38]. Corneal ulcers, bacterial keratitis, erosion syndrome, and traumatic iritis are among the complications that can occur with corneal abrasions [46].

Antibiotics can help prevent bacterial infections in corneal abrasions which, in severe cases, can cause blindness [41, 45].

10.5.4 Retinal Detachments

Traumatic retinal detachment occurs during and immediately after a blunt force is applied. The kinetic energy surpasses the tensile strength that holds the retinal and causes the retina to detach [47]. Some symptoms of retinal detachment include blurred vision, floaters, flashes of light, and a feeling of a curtain in front of the eye. Any complaints of floaters or dark shadow must be considered retinal detachment and must be evaluated by an ophthalmologist. The ophthalmic examination, after pre-dilation, should include assessments of visual acuity, pupillary responses, visual field function, and measurement of intraocular pressure. This should then be followed by an extensive slit lamp examination of the anterior segment. The affected eye should be dilated, and a fundus examination should be performed to observe the structures in the posterior segment of the eye.

Retina tears can be treated by photocoagulation and cryopexy. During photocoagulation, ophthalmologists use a laser to provide bursts of energy to the retina tissue surrounding the tear which forms clots and allows the retina to attach to the scar tissue. Cryopexy is a form of cryotherapy that is used to freeze the retinal tear to prevent further progression of the tear. Retinal detachments may require more complex surgical procedures (e.g., scleral buckle, pars plana vitrectomy, air-fluid gas exchange, silicone oil).

10.5.5 Orbital Fracture

The eyeball sits in a socket that is surrounded by thin bones that can fracture due to trauma. There are two theories that describe the mechanism of an orbital fracture: hydraulic and buckling. Hydraulic theory states that hydraulic pressure is transmitted to the thin orbital walls causing a fracture, whereas the buckling theory states force is transmitted from the rigid infraorbital rim to the thin walls causing it to fracture ("buckle") [39]. Despite the differences in the theories, the fundamental mechanism is that the force applied to the periocular region is transferred to the orbital bones causing a fracture. Both of the mechanisms are valid; however, they each cause different symptoms. For example, fractures that occur through the hydraulic mechanism usually present with symptoms such as enophthalmos [39].

In rare cases, blowout fractures (Fig. 10.4) can be a result of both of these mechanisms making the fractures quite severe. Some symptoms include diplopia on vertical gaze and pain. If the fracture entraps soft tissues or nerves, it can lead to symptoms such as bradycardia, nausea, and reduced sensation. CT scans are often preferred to diagnose the fracture and any herniation or entrapment of the structures

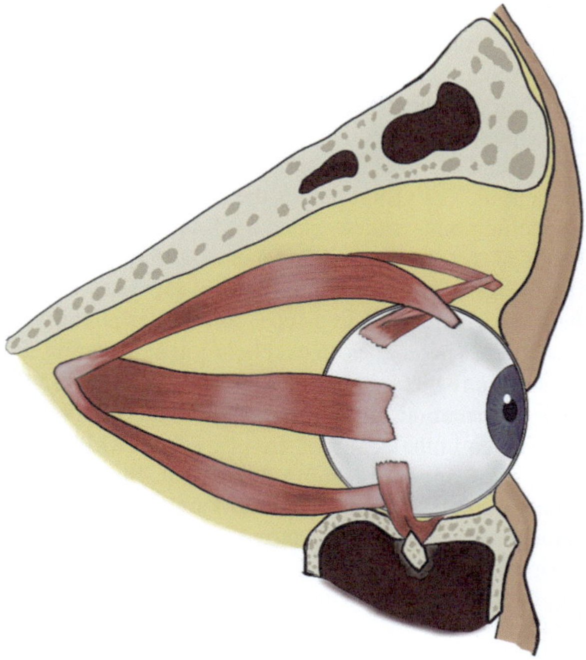

Fig. 10.4 Orbital floor fracture. (Figure by authors)

surrounding it. The fractures usually resolve without intervention in about 2 weeks, but in cases of severe entrapment, surgical treatment may be required.

10.6 Vision in Combat Sports

The reaction time (including eye-hand coordination) of a fighter is one of the most difficult skills to acquire, train, and develop [49]. The importance of reaction time can determine whether a fighter wins or loses a fight. Reaction time is defined as the time it takes to respond to a visual, auditory, or tactile stimulus [49].Training, especially at a younger age, is essential to develop an efficient visuomotor system. Between 3 and 5 years of age, the visual perceptual function improves significantly, and by the time an individual is between the ages of 7 and 9, their visual perceptual function becomes stable [50]. Improved visual function correlates with improved outcomes in goal-oriented movement similar to those seen in combat sports. The patterns of eye movement between a trained fighter and a non-trained fighter are different. Experts fixate on fewer visual points for a longer duration than non-experts and they typically have an earlier saccade [51]. Saccades are defined as rapid eye movements between different points within a visual field, usually to look at the object of interest. Saccadic movements play a crucial role in a fighter's ability to fixate on significant cues during a fight. Professional athletes frequently fixate on void spaces that are intermediary points which convey significant information [52]. Experts generally fixate their gaze centrally on the head and chest of the opponent [53]. Accurate identification and interpretation of the cues allow the fighter to predict their opponent's moves. This allows the fighter to efficiently dodge strikes from the opponent or effectively strike the opponent.

Further, the field of vision allows the fighter to gather relevant information during a fight. The visual field is the entire area that is visible when the gaze is fixed at a specific point. Athletes need a 30- to 40-degree radius to be able to visualize both hands of the opponent simultaneously [53]. In combat sports, the distance between the fighters is often minimal which decreases the visual field. The smaller visual field thus increases the critical role of peripheral vision in gathering information. Peripheral vision does an excellent job at detecting motion which allows the fighter to detect any incoming strikes from the opponent [54]. Professional boxers perceive their information differently than non-professional such that professionals fixated their fovea in the center of the visual field while utilizing their peripheral vision to track their opponent's limb movement. Similar differences can be seen in other combat sports such as judo and karate [55]. Avoiding opponent strikes prevents injuries and losses while providing an opportunity to counter attack. The use of peripheral vision despite the limited visual field in combat sports can be the deciding factor between a win and a loss.

Participants in combat sports are frequently engaged in active motion throughout the fight. Some of the motions include moving around the fighting platform for better positioning, avoiding strikes or takedowns, or moving to expose the opponent. The ability to see and recognize objects in motion or while the head is in motion and the object is static is called dynamic visual acuity (DVA). A close relationship has been established between DVA and the level of expertise in various sports [56]. Efficient DVA allows the action to be close to the fovea while still allowing maximal perception. Smooth pursuit is utilized while tracking the object to reduce motion blur. Another characteristic of vision related to DVA is the minimum position error (MPE). The concept of MPE pertains to the accuracy of the alignment of gaze to the moving object [56]. Another component that complements smooth pursuit is saccades. Smooth pursuit without saccades is usually for predicted movement. However, when an unexpected movement occurs, changes in velocity and direction of the object require smooth pursuit and saccades to keep the object in focus [57]. Efficient use of DVA and associated eye movements enables fighters to track strikes and take down attempts, defensive movements, and counter-attacks.

Another system that plays a critical role in eye movement is the vestibular-ocular system through the vestibular-ocular reflex (VOR). The vestibular system functions to maintain balance, spatial orientation, eye movements, coordination, and postural control. The oculomotor system controls include eye movements, such as saccades, smooth-pursuits, and point fixation. Both of these systems work together to ensure a smooth and stable image is transmitted to the brain. VOR is involved in controlling the stability of gaze during movement to ensure that the image is on the fovea. VOR consists of three components: the eye muscles, vestibular system, and a central processing mechanism. A deficiency in VOR correlates with disturbance in visual acuity, commonly seen in athletes with a concussion [58]. Combat sports are filled with unpredictable various body movements including ducking, weaving, striking, and grappling. These movements activate the VOR because they require the movement of the head in different directions and at different heights.

In summary, multiple visual afferent and efferent subsystems work to allow a fighter to have a clear view of their opponent. These subsystems work together in various capacities depending on the situation; however, scarce literature exists on the involvement of the ocular system in combat sports. As combat sports gain more popularity and technology advances, the opportunity for more studies increases. Additional research will improve both medical outcomes for and the performance of combat sport athletes.

10.7 Future Direction

The research on eye injuries in combat sports is both limited and outdated. Many existing studies date back several decades and have not kept pace with the evolution of these sports. Recent advancements have introduced new techniques and moves that could lead to more severe injuries. Furthermore, the field of fitness science has evolved significantly, potentially changing the nature of sports-related injuries. Therefore, conducting contemporary research on ocular injuries in combat sports could be highly valuable. Leveraging current technological and medical advancements could provide a solid basis for collecting up-to-date data. This information is crucial for enhancing the safety of athletes by improving the sport itself and designing more effective protective gear to reduce the incidence of injuries.

10.8 Conclusion

Combat sports, among the earliest forms of athletic competition, serve various purposes and inherently pose a risk of injuries to different body parts, including the head, face, torso, and limbs. The ocular system, in particular, is vulnerable, mainly due to its anatomical position and the frequency of facial targeting in these sports. Common ocular injuries in combat sports include eyebrow and eyelid lacerations, hyphema, corneal abrasions, retinal detachments, and orbital fractures. It is crucial to understand the mechanisms behind these injuries for effective management and prevention of complications. This understanding can also inform the development of safety-enhancing rules and regulations. Additionally, focusing on the ocular system in combat sports opens up research opportunities regarding the role of vision in athletic performance. Exploring how athletes can optimally use their vision could provide a competitive edge leading to success. Hence, there is a significant need for research on the ocular system's involvement in combat sports, which could further advance the fields of sports, sports science, and medicine.

References

1. Dellinger B. The oldest sport. Natl Wrestl Hall Fame. https://nwhof.org/national-wrestling-hall-of-fame/pages/the-oldest-sport
2. Zazryn TR. A 16 year study of injuries to professional boxers in the state of Victoria, Australia. Br J Sports Med. 2003;37(4):321–4. https://doi.org/10.1136/bjsm.37.4.321.
3. Lambert C, Ritzmann R, Lambert S, et al. Prevalence of sport injuries in Olympic combat sports: a cross-sectional study examining one Olympic period. J Sports Med Phys Fitness. 2022;62(11):1496. https://doi.org/10.23736/S0022-4707.22.13334-7.
4. Jordan BD, Campbell EA. Acute injuries among professional boxers in New York State: a two-year survey. Phys Sportsmed. 1988;16(1):87–91. https://doi.org/10.1080/00913847.1988.11709407.
5. Barbieri FA, Rodrigues ST. Editorial: the role of eye movements in sports and active living. Front Sports Act Living. 2020;2:603206. https://doi.org/10.3389/fspor.2020.603206.
6. Williams AM, Davids K, Williams JGP. Visual perception and action in sport. E & FN Spon; 1999.
7. Myers RJ, Linakis SW, Mello MJ, Linakis JG. Competitive wrestling-related injuries in school aged athletes in U.S. Emergency Departments. West J Emerg Med. 2010;11(5):442–9.
8. Jarrett GJ, Orwin JF, Dick RW. Injuries in collegiate wrestling. Am J Sports Med. 1998;26(5):674–80. https://doi.org/10.1177/03635465980260051301.
9. Stanbouly D, Murphy R, Murphy TX, McDoniell J, Lee KC, Chuang SK. Craniomaxillofacial injuries from the sport of wrestling: a query of the National Electronic Injury Surveillance System (NEISS). Oral Maxillofac Surg. 2021;26(3):393–400. https://doi.org/10.1007/s10006-021-01004-3.
10. Powell JW. National athletic injury/illness reporting system: eye injuries in college wrestling. Int Ophthalmol Clin. 1981;21(4):47–58. https://doi.org/10.1097/00004397-198102140-00005.
11. Forrest LA, Schuller DE, Strauss RH. Management of orbital blow-out fractures: case reports and discussion. Am J Sports Med. 1989;17(2):217–20. https://doi.org/10.1177/036354658901700211.
12. Holland EJ, Mahanti RL, Belongia EA, et al. Ocular involvement in an outbreak of herpes gladiatorum. Am J Ophthalmol. 1992;114(6):680–4. https://doi.org/10.1016/S0002-9394(14)74044-9.
13. Zare Mehrjardi MA, Eye Research Center, Farabi Eye Hospital, Tehran University of Medical Sciences, Zare Mehrjardi H, et al. Corneal Ectasis among wrestlers: report of two cases. Ann Appl Sport Sci. 2014;2(2):23–8. https://doi.org/10.18869/acadpub.aassjournal.2.2.23.
14. Boddy K. Boxing: a cultural history. Reaktion Books; 2013.
15. Siewe J, Rudat J, Zarghooni K, et al. Injuries in competitive boxing. A prospective study. Int J Sports Med. 2014;36(03):249–53. https://doi.org/10.1055/s-0034-1387764.
16. Brown DA, Leung FT, Evans K, Grant G, Hides JA. Vestibular and oculomotor function in male combat sport athletes. J Sci Med Sport. 2022;25(6):524–8. https://doi.org/10.1016/j.jsams.2022.02.004.
17. Bledsoe GH, Li G, Levy F. Injury risk in professional boxing. South Med J. 2005;98(10):994–8. https://doi.org/10.1097/01.smj.0000182498.19288.e2.
18. Potter MR, Snyder AJ, Smith GA. Boxing injuries presenting to U.S. Emergency Departments, 1990–2008. Am J Prev Med. 2011;40(4):462–7. https://doi.org/10.1016/j.amepre.2010.12.018.
19. Banman CJ, Schneider KJ, Cluff T, Peters RM. Altered vestibular balance function in combat sport athletes. J Neurotrauma. 2021;38(16):2291–300. https://doi.org/10.1089/neu.2020.7432.
20. Jones NP. Eye injury in sport. Sports Med. 1989;7(3):163–81. https://doi.org/10.2165/00007256-198907030-00003.
21. Wedrich A, Velikay M, Binder S, Radax U, Stolba U, Datlinger P. Ocular findings in asymptomatic amateur boxers. Retina. 1993;13(2):114–9. https://doi.org/10.1097/00006982-199313020-00004.

22. Vadalà G, Mollo M, Roberto S, Fea A. Boxing and the eyes: morphological aspects of the ocular system in boxers. Eur J Ophthalmol. 1997;7(2):174–80. https://doi.org/10.1177/112067219700700210.
23. Giovinazzo VJ, Yannuzzi LA, Sorenson JA, Delrowe DJ, Cambell EA. The ocular complications of boxing. Ophthalmology. 1987;94(6):587–96. https://doi.org/10.1016/S0161-6420(87)33404-9.
24. Kordi R, editor. Combat sports medicine. Springer; 2009.
25. Bianco M, Vaiano AS, Colella F, et al. Ocular complications of boxing. Br J Sports Med. 2005;39(2):70. https://doi.org/10.1136/bjsm.2003.006643.
26. Maguire JI. Retinal injury and detachment in boxers. JAMA J Am Med Assoc. 1986;255(18):2451. https://doi.org/10.1001/jama.1986.03370180077035.
27. Shere JL, Boole JR, Holtel MR, Amoroso PJ. An analysis of 3599 midfacial and 1141 orbital blowout fractures among 4426 United States Army Soldiers, 1980–2000. Otolaryngol Neck Surg. 2004;130(2):164–70. https://doi.org/10.1016/j.otohns.2003.09.018.
28. Beck KD, Hernandez L. Central retinal artery occlusion in a 21-year-old boxer. Ophthalmology. 2015;122(8):1568. https://doi.org/10.1016/j.ophtha.2015.05.018.
29. Seungmo K, Greenwell C, Damon A, Lee J, Mahony D. An analysis of spectator motives in an individual combat sport: a study of mixed martial arts fans. Sport Mark Q. 2008;17:109–19.
30. Lystad RP, Gregory K, Wilson J. The epidemiology of injuries in mixed martial arts: a systematic review and meta-analysis. Orthop J Sports Med. 2014;2(1):2325967113518492. https://doi.org/10.1177/2325967113518492.
31. Bishop SH, La Bounty P, Devlin M. Mixed martial arts: a comprehensive review. J Sport Hum Perform. 2013;1(1) https://doi.org/10.12922/jshp.v1i1.6.
32. Buse GJ. No holds barred sport fighting: a 10 year review of mixed martial arts competition. Br J Sports Med. 2006;40(2):169–72. https://doi.org/10.1136/bjsm.2005.021295.
33. Hutchison MG, Lawrence DW, Cusimano MD, Schweizer TA. Head trauma in mixed martial arts. Am J Sports Med. 2014;42(6):1352–8. https://doi.org/10.1177/0363546514526151.
34. Brown DA, Grant G, Evans K, Leung FT, Hides JA. Evaluation of the vestibular/ocular motor screening assessment in active combat sport athletes: an exploratory study. Brain Inj. 2022;36(8):961–7. https://doi.org/10.1080/02699052.2022.2109741.
35. Rainey CE. Determining the prevalence and assessing the severity of injuries in mixed martial arts athletes. N Am J Sports Phys Ther NAJSPT. 2009;4(4):190–9.
36. Fliotsos MJ, Reed DS, Giles G, et al. Prevalence, patterns, and characteristics of eye injuries in professional mixed martial arts. Clin Ophthalmol Auckl NZ. 2021;15:2759–66. https://doi.org/10.2147/OPTH.S319025.
37. Bledsoe GH, Hsu EB, Grabowski JG, Brill JD, Li G. Incidence of injury in professional mixed martial arts competitions. J Sports Sci Med. 2006;5(CSSI):136–42.
38. Ahmed F, House RJ, Feldman BH. Corneal abrasions and corneal foreign bodies. Prim Care Clin Off Pract. 2015;42(3):363–75. https://doi.org/10.1016/j.pop.2015.05.004.
39. Gart MS, Gosain AK. Evidence-based medicine: orbital floor fractures. Plast Reconstr Surg. 2014;134(6):1345–55. https://doi.org/10.1097/PRS.0000000000000719.
40. Pierce JD, Reinbold KA, Lyngard BC, Goldman RJ, Pastore CM. Direct measurement of punch force during six professional boxing matches. J Quant Anal Sports. 2006;2(2) https://doi.org/10.2202/1559-0410.1004.
41. Corrales G, Curreri A. Eye trauma in boxing. Clin Sports Med. 2009;28(4):591–607. https://doi.org/10.1016/j.csm.2009.07.004.
42. Ko AC, Satterfield KR, Korn BS, Kikkawa DO. Eyelid and periorbital soft tissue trauma. Facial Plast Surg Clin N Am. 2017;25(4):605–16. https://doi.org/10.1016/j.fsc.2017.06.011.
43. Walton W, Von Hagen S, Grigorian R, Zarbin M. Management of traumatic hyphema. Surv Ophthalmol. 2002;47(4):297–334. https://doi.org/10.1016/S0039-6257(02)00317-X.
44. Chen K. Hyphema. Medscape.
45. Wilson SA, Last A. Management of corneal abrasions. Am Fam Physician. 2004;70(1):123–8.

46. Domingo E, Moshirfar M, Zabbo CP. Corneal abrasion. In: StatPearls. StatPearls Publishing; 2023. http://www.ncbi.nlm.nih.gov/books/NBK532960/. Accessed 14 Dec 2023.
47. Olsen TW, Chang TS, Sternberg P. Retinal detachments associated with blunt trauma. Semin Ophthalmol. 1995;10(1):17–27. https://doi.org/10.3109/08820539509059976.
48. Enoch J, McDonald L, Jones L, Jones PR, Crabb DP. Evaluating whether sight is the most valued sense. JAMA Ophthalmol. 2019;137(11):1317–20. https://doi.org/10.1001/jamaophthalmol.2019.3537.
49. Dinçer N, Kilinç Z, Ilbak I. Comparison of visual simple reaction time performances of boxers and wrestlers. Pak J Med Health Sci. 2022;16(2):467–9. https://doi.org/10.53350/pjmhs22162467.
50. Case-Smith J, editor. Occupational therapy for children. 5th ed. Elsevier Mosby; 2005.
51. Ju YY, Liu YH, Cheng CH, et al. Effects of combat training on visuomotor performance in children aged 9 to 12 years – an eye-tracking study. BMC Pediatr. 2018;18(1):39. https://doi.org/10.1186/s12887-018-1038-6.
52. Piras A, Lobietti R, Squatrito S. A study of saccadic eye movement dynamics in volleyball: comparison between athletes and non-athletes. J Sports Med Phys Fitness. 2010;50(1):99–108.
53. Krabben K, Mann D, Lojanica M, et al. How wide should you view to fight? Establishing the size of the visual field necessary for grip fighting in judo. J Sports Sci. 2022;40(2):236–47. https://doi.org/10.1080/02640414.2021.1987721.
54. Vater C, Kredel R, Hossner EJ. Examining the functionality of peripheral vision: from fundamental understandings to applied sport science. Curr Issues Sport Sci CISS. 2017;2:010. https://doi.org/10.36950/2017ciss010.
55. Kato T. Using "Enzan No Metsuke" (Gazing at the Far Mountain) as a visual search strategy in Kendo. Front Sports Act Living. 2020;2:40. https://doi.org/10.3389/fspor.2020.00040.
56. Palidis DJ, Wyder-Hodge PA, Fooken J, Spering M. Distinct eye movement patterns enhance dynamic visual acuity. PLoS One. 2017;12(2):e0172061. https://doi.org/10.1371/journal.pone.0172061.
57. De Brouwer S, Yuksel D, Blohm G, Missal M, Lefèvre P. What triggers catch-up saccades during visual tracking? J Neurophysiol. 2002;87(3):1646–50. https://doi.org/10.1152/jn.00432.2001.
58. Landers MR, Donatelli R, Nash J, Bascharon R. Evidence of dynamic visual acuity impairment in asymptomatic mixed martial arts fighters. Concussion Lond Engl. 2017;2(3):CNC41. https://doi.org/10.2217/cnc-2016-0032.

Index

E. Waisberg et al. (eds.), *Ophthalmology of Sports*,
https://doi.org/10.1007/978-3-031-88645-4

MIX
Papier aus verantwortungsvollen Quellen
Paper from responsible sources
FSC® C105338

If you have any concerns about our products,
you can contact us on
ProductSafety@springernature.com

In case Publisher is established outside the EU,
the EU authorized representative is:
Springer Nature Customer Service Center GmbH
Europaplatz 3, 69115 Heidelberg, Germany

Printed by Libri Plureos GmbH
in Hamburg, Germany